LIVING WITH
PARKINSON'S

LIVING WITH
PARKINSON'S

Gabriella Rogers

NEW
HOLLAND

In memory of my beautiful mother, Giovina

First published in 2011 by New Holland Publishers (Australia) Pty Ltd
Sydney • Auckland • London • Cape Town

www.newholland.com.au

1/66 Gibbes Street Chatswood NSW 2067 Australia
218 Lake Road Northcote Auckland New Zealand
86 Edgware Road London W2 2EA United Kingdom
80 McKenzie Street Cape Town 8001 South Africa

A record of this book is available at the National Library of Australia

ISBN 9781741108927

Publisher: Diane Jardine
Publishing manager: Lliane Clarke
Senior editor: Mary Trewby
Designer: Celeste Valok
Production manager: Olga Dementiev
Printer: McPherson's Printing Group

CONTENTS

FOREWORD

Parkinson's is an insidious disease. Living and caring for a sufferer of Parkinson's is a very difficult and challenging undertaking. My husband, Mike Leyland, travelled all over the countryside as one of the Leyland Brothers, exploring the many corners of our continent. But the journey he had with Parkinson's was one that he did not want to take. Mike lost his battle in September 2009 after complications relating to the disease.

When a friend or family member is diagnosed with Parkinson's, there are many battles that need to be tackled. Most importantly, support, love and understanding are imperative for the sufferer, the carer and the families. It is difficult to know what the sufferer is thinking and this is often not helped by the tendency to lock their thoughts up by questioning 'why is this happening to me?' As a carer, you have to be a major supporter, do a lot of encouraging and try your hardest to continue on in a normal way. This is very hard when you know that the situation is not going to ease.

Another important aspect of the battle against Parkinson's is seeking out the right advice. My daughter, Alison, discovered the Parkinson's Clinic at Concord Hospital after she herself noticed a significant deterioration in Mike's health when we returned from a holiday. This was one of the best discoveries that Mike and I could have ever made. Dr Michael Hayes, the neurologist who attended to Mike at the clinic, was an exceptional man. He always had the time to talk to you and discuss any problems. He even rang me at home on one occasion to finish telling me something we were discussing at one of our appointments. You were never rushed away and he always gave a lot of encouragement to the patient. Dr Hayes would always say 'you're doing well', knowing that everything was not the best. On Mike's passing, Dr Hayes sent a handwritten letter with his thoughts and demonstrated the true caring nature of those at the clinic.

Establishing a support network is also significant in your battle with Parkinson's and those at the hospital were always there to offer their counsel and support. Parkinson's NSW also has a wonderful support program for both carers and patients. Branches all over the state provide direct help lines, meetings and conferences, all aimed specifically at benefiting the patients and carers. Their mission to enhance the lives of those living with Parkinson's is something that I have personally experienced and I too wish to see a community free of Parkinson's.

When taking on the battle with Parkinson's, always be prepared. Seek out options for care and support well before you need them, so you are ready if required. Talk to other carers and those working with and around the disease so that you can be informed. Always consider accepting that offer of assistance when needed; looking after yourself is key to being a good carer and support person.

Living with a Parkinson's sufferer gives you many feelings, especially as you see the one you love disappearing before your eyes, especially not knowing what they are going through inside. You can only be there all the way with them and help them through this part of their life.

Support, love and lots of understanding are necessary for any illness.

Margie Leyland

1. Defining Parkinson's Disease

Dozens of health experts and people who have lived with the disease for many years were interviewed in researching this book. While their initial reaction when diagnosed is usually one of shock, their subsequent journey is much less dramatic. There are examples throughout the book of people who've lived with the disease for 20 years and who continue to climb mountains, run marathons or walk their children down the aisle. Author John Ball has lived with the disease for over half his life, and having completed a string of marathons, his motto sums up his attitude: 'I am not defined by the disease. I have Parkinson's. It doesn't have me.'

Paula Argy was diagnosed more than a decade ago. She hasn't allowed her diagnosis to destroy her dreams of having children and she speaks of the 'highs' of motherhood, which far outweigh the lows of her illness. Her days are very active with school drop offs, ballet lessons, making cupcakes and sewing costumes for her girls. Her positive attitude and the love and support of her friends and family have certainly enabled her to deal with any challenges along the way.

While the disease affects tens of thousands of Australians, many people only know Parkinson's disease as something that gives you 'the shakes'. But neurologist Victor Fung says 20 to 30 per cent of people who have the disease won't experience signs of shaking: 'If they don't shake, it might come to them as a surprise that they have Parkinson's.'

The diagnosis of American actor Michael J. Fox and his public declaration in 1998 put Parkinson's disease in the spotlight. The actor noticed a twitch in his little finger, which was the first real sign of trouble. It was while he was filming *Doc Hollywood*, which was released in 1991. It wasn't until seven years later that he revealed to the world that he had Parkinson's. He was 37 when he told *People* magazine: 'It's not that I had a deep, dark secret. It was just my thing to deal with ... I think I can help people by talking.' A few years after declaring his private struggle, he launched a research foundation to raise funds and increase awareness. In his latest memoir, *Always Looking Up*, he describes paralysed actor Christopher Reeve and cyclist and cancer survivor Lance Armstrong as his role models. 'Each had taken a negative and turned it into a positive. I didn't have to let the terms of a disease define me—I could redefine the terms. And maybe in the process get a better deal for me and everyone else in my situation.'[1]

> *It seems strange to say it, but I had to learn to respect Parkinson's disease. Instead of being reactive, I started being proactive, reading all the materials available, meeting with doctors, surgeons, researchers, and finally, after many years of lingering fear, getting to know fellow Parkinson's patients and other members of the community.*[2]
>
> —Michael J Fox

What is Parkinson's disease?

Parkinson's disease was named after English doctor James Parkinson in 1817. He wrote numerous medical books, but was famous for 'An essay on the shaking palsy', which established Parkinson's disease as a recognised medical condition. His essay was based on six cases he had either met at his own practice or seen during walks in his neighbourhood. He hoped writing the essay would encourage others to study the condition.

The French neurologist, Jean-Martin Charcot, who fully recognised the significance of James Parkinson's work 60 years
after he had described it as the 'shaking palsy', gave the disease
its name.[3] Charcot also added new features to the list of symptoms, and began a study into the many facets of Parkinson's
disease. The study continues to the present day, and over the
past few years the list of potential problems has grown. Sleep
disturbances, including nightmares, have been identified as a
feature of the disease.

Parkinson's disease affects millions of people around the
world, and in Australia more than 80,000 people have been
diagnosed with the disease.[4] It's a condition that strikes the central nervous system and causes involuntary tremor, stiffness, slow
movement and loss of balance. In Australia, it's the second most
common neurodegenerative disease after Alzheimer's disease.

The nervous system is made up of cells called neurons that
specialise in transmitting electrical nerve impulses and carry
information from one part of the body to another.[5] In Parkinson's disease, neurons in the mid section of the brain (substantia nigra) gradually die or become impaired. This leads to a loss
of dopamine, which is a chemical that stimulates nerve cells to
control the muscles and helps with movement.

> *Dopamine is more like engine oil than petrol. Without*
> *dopamine you can still move, but the movements are*
> *corrupted. They become slow or stiff. That's what gives rise*
> *to the symptoms of Parkinson's disease.*
>
> —Dr Victor Fung, neurologist

Studies have shown that most patients have lost 60 to 80 per
cent, or more, of the dopamine-producing cells in the substantia nigra by the time symptoms appear.[6]

This loss of dopamine is the key to providing some of the
most effective therapies for Parkinson's disease, with drugs that

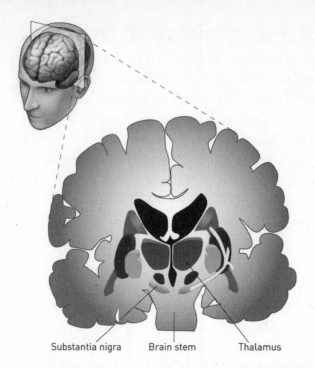

Substantia nigra   Brain stem   Thalamus

In Parkinson's disease, the neurons in the mid-section of the brain (substantia nigra) gradually die or become impaired. This leads to a loss of dopamine, a chemical that stimulates nerve cells to control the muscles and helps with movement.

may 'look like' dopamine (dopamine agonists) or drugs that the body can transform into dopamine (L-dopa). These medications typically produce a dramatic response to the movement problems and people may feel like they're returning to a 'normal life'. This is known as the honeymoon period, and can last for many years.

Many people with Parkinson's disease will only experience movement problems. Over time, movement can become less stable despite medication, and other issues not relating to mobility may become more pronounced.

Professor Malcolm Horne, of Melbourne's Florey Neuroscience Institutes, says while dopamine has an important role in Parkinson's disease and causes the initial (predominantly movement) symptoms, neurons in other parts of the brain that do not use the chemical dopamine are also affected. These neurons help control the gut, bladder, blood pressure and sleep cycle. When neurons in the cortex are disturbed many people get hallucinations and dementia. It is these neurons that make the disease untreatable and put people in nursing homes.

Doctors know a lot about what happens to the brain in someone who has Parkinson's disease, and scientists have discovered some important clues to the causes, and in some cases treatment. They are learning more about the genetics of the disease and they know roughly where the trouble is. 'But we still don't know how to use these clues to find the solution,' says Professor Horne.

That means that at present there are no treatments to halt or slow the disease. The therapies currently available to patients can only help relieve the symptoms.

Who gets Parkinson's and why?

The *Oxford Medical Dictionary* says the disease is associated with ageing. That's partly true, because age is a major risk factor, and the symptoms progress as the person gets older. Features of the disease commonly vary between young and old people. The average age of diagnosis is 65 years, but one in seven people diagnosed with the disease is under the age of 45.[7] Parkinson's disease affects a large group of people of working age and many are forced to change jobs or give up their careers as movement and cognitive problems start to affect their daily lives.

> *The youngest person diagnosed in Australia with Parkinson's disease is 14 years old.*
> —HTA, *Help for Today: Hope for Tomorrow*

The disease does not discriminate between male and female—both sexes are equally likely to suffer from Parkinson's disease. Nor does it target any particular ethnic group.

Scientists have not been able to work out why some people develop the illness and others do not. Only about 10 per cent of people diagnosed will have another close relative affected, but a strong family history of genetic mutation is extremely rare.[8]

More than half of the patients who develop the disease before the age of 20 have a defect in a gene called parkin and they respond remarkably well to small doses of medication to increase levels of dopamine in the brain. Both parents would have to carry the faulty parkin gene to pass it onto one of their children (a recessive gene).

In some rare cases among families, mutations of another gene called SNCA can predispose a person to Parkinson's disease. It was the first gene found to have an association with the illness. If one parent has Parkinson's because they have a faulty copy of this gene, each of his or her children has a 50 per cent chance of inheriting the mutation.[9]

Professor Horne says the SNCA gene makes the protein alpha-synuclein. Alpha-synuclein is a major component in the Lewy Body in dopamine cells in the brain tissue, which is a hallmark sign of the disease. This means that alpha-synuclein is important in the development of Parkinson's disease, even if you don't have a mutation in the gene.

Research suggests that a cell's protein disposal system isn't working in people with Parkinson's disease, and this can lead to a harmful build-up of abnormal or damaged proteins and can cause cells to die. Other studies have found evidence of clumps of protein that have developed inside the brain cells of people with Parkinson's disease, and that may contribute to the death of neurons.[10] They accumulate within the cell to form the Lewy Body, which was identified by Dr Friedrich Lewy in 1912. These microscopic protein deposits disturb the brain's normal functioning, and the body's failure to dispose of alpha-synuclein may be the root cause of Parkinson's disease, which has prompted researchers around the world to investigate this phenomenon.

It is also suggested that inflammation or over-stimulation of cells (because of toxins or other factors) may play a role in the development of the disease.[11]

The parkin and SNCA genes are not the only ones to be identified as having a role in inherited forms of Parkinson's disease. The others include DJ1, PINK1 and LRRK2.[12]

Professor Garth Nicholson, a Sydney neurogeneticist, says several known mutations can be picked up in genetic testing. While these tests are available commercially, they cost about $6000; because they don't alter the course of managing the disease, they are not routinely performed. It's hoped new technology will make genetic testing more affordable in the near future (this will be discussed further in Chapter 7).

There is a theory that environmental factors are partly to blame for Parkinson's disease, as with many other chronic diseases. Factors such as exposure to pesticides and herbicides have been linked to increased risk.[13] Karen Rowland from Perth believes she developed the disease after she was exposed to the chemical DDT as a child, when she was growing up in the mining town of Kalgoorlie. DDT was widely used to control pests in Australian agriculture in the 1950s, but was banned in 1987.[14]

Professor Horne says anecdotal evidence suggests a relatively higher incidence of people diagnosed with Parkinson's disease in Victoria's Goulburn Valley, where crop spraying is prevalent.

> *We know that people who've had a lifelong increased exposure to environmental insecticide seem to have a higher risk. What we don't know is how that plays out with some genes. If your genetic make-up is that you're not very good at breaking down toxins you might be more susceptible. So it's not definitive that environmental factors are to blame, but there are strong reasons to suggest they increase risk.*
> —Professor Malcolm Horne, Florey Neuroscience Institutes

A number of toxins, such as 1-methyl-4-phenyl-1,2,3,6-tetrahy-
dropyridine, or MPTP (found in some forms of synthetic heroin), can cause Parkinson's-like symptoms in humans.[15] The first
case of MPTP-induced Parkinson's disease happened in 1976
after a student took synthetic heroin: within several days he had
developed severe symptoms of the disease. Although patients
affected by the toxin show all the clinical features of Parkinson's
disease, it's not the same. MPTP-induced symptoms develop rapidly, over a number of days, whereas Parkinson's disease develops
spontaneously and progresses slowly from onset to end stage.[16]

Viruses could also be a possible trigger for Parkinson's
disease, but experts believe it is more likely that some viruses
can damage the same part of the brain that degenerates in
people with Parkinson's. For example, some people developed
encephalopathy (brain dysfunction) after the 1918 Spanish flu
epidemic, which claimed an estimated 50 million lives world-
wide. Those who had encephalopathy developed severe, progressive, Parkinson's-like symptoms. A group of Taiwanese women
showed similar signs after contracting herpes virus infections.
In these women, the Parkinson's-like symptoms, which later
disappeared, were linked to a temporary inflammation of the
substantia nigra in the brain.[17]

Several lines of research suggest free radicals (minute chemical particles) play a role in the disease's development. Free
radicals can cause cell damage—triggered by environmental
and dietary factors such as cigarette smoke, pollution, radiation
and fatty foods. The damage is often referred to as oxidative
stress, which causes a breakdown of DNA, proteins and fats,[18]
and it has been detected in the brains of affected patients.

Ironically, there's also evidence that smoking has a protective effect. 'I would have thought people who smoked would
have more chance of free radical damage, so it goes against
that,' says Professor Garth Nicholson. Neurologist Michael
Hayes says the protection from smoking is unlikely to come

from the nicotine, keeping in mind that the effect is only very small compared with the detrimental effect of smoking on other areas of the body. 'You wouldn't encourage people to smoke because it statistically reduces the risk of Parkinson's disease.'

The region of the brain involved in Parkinson's disease is very electrically active, placing demands on the cell's energy production and increasing oxidative stress. Neurologist Dr Scott Whyte says a particular calcium channel found in these cells is an important factor. A variety of recent studies has suggested that altering the activity of these cell channels may alter disease progression (dietary calcium intake has not been implicated in this and calcium supplements should continue to be taken if required). It is too early to know how successful this theory will be, but this is an example of the importance of basic scientific research in understanding the disease and driving therapy.

How is Parkinson's diagnosed?

Many people who have symptoms of the disease are misdiagnosed. The problem is that there is no definitive test to identify a patient suffering from Parkinson's disease. Neurologist Dr Victor Fung says a general practitioner usually has an idea that something is wrong, and that it might be Parkinson's disease, but would want to confirm the diagnosis with a specialist.

A neurologist will pore over a patient's medical history to pick vital clues in the form of classic symptoms. For example, if a person has experienced a shake for eight months and it has been getting worse, a neurologist will know very quickly whether it's related to the disease.

> *Someone with Parkinson's disease would usually experience tremor, even when their hands are resting and not doing anything.*
>
> —Dr Victor Fung

There is a fair chance that someone might not have the disease if they experience tremor only when using their hands or limbs. A tremor doesn't necessarily begin in the hands. It can affect the arms, legs, jaw or face.

The disease usually affects one side of the body, especially during the early stages. Patients often complain of stiffness in the limbs and the trunk of the body. A neurologist will ask various questions, such as the following.

- Do you have trouble walking?
- Do you have problems turning in bed?
- Is it hard to get out of a chair?
- Is driving becoming more difficult?
- Do you drag your leg while walking?

A person with Parkinson's disease usually experiences slow movement, and spontaneous movement becomes more difficult. This can be devastating for the patient who starts to struggle with simple tasks, reducing their independence.

Gradually, a patient's posture becomes less stable, and their balance and coordination become impaired. Their posture takes on a stooped appearance and they develop a forward or backward lean.

This makes it more likely for a patient to fall and suffer an injury (preventing falls is further discussed in Chapter 5). In the later stages of the disease, walking may also be affected. People with Parkinson's disease may halt in mid-stride or may walk with a series of small, quick steps as if hurrying forward to keep their balance.[19]

> *Brian's never really had a shake. His shake was internal, in that he could feel all his organs inside shaking.*
>
> —Pauline England, aged 73, wife and carer
> of a Parkinson's disease patient

*I don't have external tremor but I have one inside. Feels like
my arm is vibrating on the inside.*
    —Karen Rowland, diagnosed with Parkinson's in her 40s

Ruling out other conditions

*If you give them dopamine and it doesn't do anything for them,
it begs the question whether the diagnosis is correct.*
    —Dr Michael Hayes, neurologist

Neurologist Michael Hayes says if people are showing out-ward signs of the disease but aren't responsive to dopamine medication, then their diagnosis should be reviewed. Studies have shown that up to a quarter of patients with Parkinson's symptoms are given another diagnosis. For example, multiple system atrophy is a rapidly progressive disease, which bears similar features to Parkinson's but the initial signs are different. People with this type of atrophy (degeneration of cells) usually have problems with bladder control and suffer from dizziness and impotence.

Progressive supranuclear palsy is a disorder that af-fects a different part of the brain. In the first year people often lose their balance and fall. The telltale feature of this disorder is a loss of eye movement and the inability to gaze vertically.

Essential tremor is another condition that can be confused with Parkinson's disease. It usually causes trembling of the hands during use, but the tremor reduces significantly or stops altogether when the hands are resting. The hands, head and voice are often affected, and there is commonly a family history of tremor.[20] Occasionally people with Parkinson's dis-ease may develop a tremor while resting and moving, making the distinction from essential tremor more difficult.

What are the symptoms of Parkinson's?

People with Parkinson's disease don't always share the same symptoms, and varied symptoms may respond differently to medication. This partly explains the range of presentations and therapy regimes of patients with Parkinson's disease. This is a general guide of the signs to look for.[21] These features commonly affect one side of the body more than the other in the initial stages:

- tremor (shaking), typically when limbs are resting
- rigidity (muscle stiffness) that can produce pain from not moving
- bradykinesia, or slowness in voluntary movement, such as standing up, walking and sitting down
- balance problems—the loss of reflexes affects the posture and falling is common
- 'Parkinson's gait'—the typical walk includes shuffling, drooped shoulders, lack of arm swing, head facing down, and leaning backwards or forwards unnaturally; patients find it difficult to start walking, and steps become smaller and slower
- micrographia—small handwriting
- lethargy and depression.

Other symptoms

> *It's a great idea to keep a diary if someone wants to learn about their symptoms. But we don't want them to become dependent on it, because life then becomes a recording of every problem.*
> —Margarita Makoutonina, occupational therapist

One of the most prevalent symptoms among Parkinson's patients is the loss of smell, and 70 to 90 per cent of patients are affected. It's also thought that loss of smell may present much earlier than motor deficits.[22] If that's the case, it will be a valuable tool in early diagnosis, before other symptoms take hold. (This is further discussed in Chapter 7.)

Changes in sleep (REM behavioural sleep disorder) have more recently been linked to Parkinson's disease. The problem can precede the onset of more typical features, often by many years. This can occur when a person experiences more vivid dreams and restlessness or thrashing about.

Mental health issues can develop as a result of the disease or because of the side effects of medication. This topic is becoming better understood, as more recognition is given to problems of gambling and compulsive behaviour.

Depression affects at least half of all patients at some stage of their illness. Depression often stems from the grief of being diagnosed, the lack of mobility, the loss of independence and the inability to take control. Depression may also be caused by other chemical changes occurring within the brain. Antidepressants might be necessary for more severe cases. Others who experience mild forms of depression will benefit from counselling and exercise.

Anxiety is also common, and it can be accompanied by feelings of restlessness, apprehension and irritability. If these feelings occur during periods where medication isn't effective, the motor fluctuations need to be treated aggressively.[23] People can experience fluctuations during the day because they're not achieving a stable response with their medication as the disease progresses. (Refer to Chapter 4: Stages of Parkinson's.)

Visual hallucinations are more frequent when someone has lived with the disease for five to ten years, and when they have developed the disease at an older age. Hallucinations can be caused by the disease itself and made worse by the medications in someone who is susceptible. Neurologist Dr Victor Fung says about 30 per cent of people with Parkinson's will develop hallucinations at some stage throughout their illness, with the hallucinations often worsening as the amount of medication is increased. Not all hallucinations are worrying and need treatment, but when they become distressing or result in abnormal behaviour, treatment is required. Part of the solution may be to change the type of medications used, or reduce the dose. If these simple approaches are not sufficient, then specific antipsychotic medication may be required.

Short-term memory can be affected even in the early stages of the disease. Dementia usually develops after at least 10 to 15 years of the illness in older-onset patients, and after 20 to 25 years of illness in younger-onset patients. Hallucinations are often the first signs of dementia, and confusion can become the next sign to manifest. Hallucinations may also result from other illnesses, such as infections, and they should be considered if hallucinations occur or worsen. The cause may not be Parkinson's disease and a review by a GP may be required.

Freezing occurs when a patient feels like their feet are glued to the ground. It often happens while walking through doorways. It can lead to falls. Advice from a physiotherapist can be helpful in developing ways of tackling the problem of freezing. (This topic is discussed further in Chapter 5.)

Peter McWilliam from Pennant Hills was diagnosed with Parkinson's disease at the age of 50 in 1992. 'I was getting terribly tired,' he said.

> *I began to develop facial masking—when your face can't express emotion very easily—and my walking had become a bit clumsy, a bit too clumsy. My left arm wouldn't swing. I put that down to old football injuries. From that point on, things began to gradually worsen. I lost my sense of smell and back spasms set in. At that stage I hadn't developed the telltale tremor.*

Peter went to see many doctors to complain about his shoulder, which felt stiff. A rheumatologist considered him too young to have Parkinson's disease, even though he displayed some of the symptoms. Eventually Peter sought a referral from his GP.

'I went to the public library to get a textbook on it and there it was. A perfect description of me in the early days of Parkinson's disease. I was wandering around for a few months before I saw a neurologist,' he said.

Peter said he had become a hypochondriac, until he was formally diagnosed. 'There's no test for the disease at all. The neurologist just uses his experience. They give you an MRI [brain scan] to eliminate other potential problems like a tumour or stroke.'

> *I found my diagnosis a relief ... finally there was something to explain problems I'd been experiencing all those years.*
> —Peter McWilliam

Karen Rowland from Perth wasn't diagnosed for two years after experiencing her first symptoms. 'My left arm didn't swing, which I ignored until I started to drag my left foot, and when I went to my GP I had every test you could imagine,' she said. 'I had scans, I went to the physiotherapist, I did everything, but no one could find anything. So my GP sent me to a neurologist to rule everything out. I went on my own, thinking I would get the all-clear.'

When Karen was diagnosed with the disease at the age of 47, her neurologist gave her little information. He just said if you take your medication, no one will know for years:

> *I was shocked. I made an error of judgment because I decided not to tell anybody. I just told my immediate family I had a neurological condition and that medication would fix it.*

Karen kept her secret for three years. She believes the cognitive changes were the most disabling part of her condition.

She ran a successful conveyancing business until her symptoms caught up with her.

'My thinking was getting slower and I couldn't get my mail organised and do ten things at once. I wasn't hopeless, but I wasn't up to my usual standard at work,' she says. Karen had to quit her job and believes others have been forced to do the same because of their impaired performance.

'A lot of people think it's not going to happen to them and it does. I know of a bank manager who has taken up a cleaning business. I think most people with Parkinson's have cognitive problems.'

You'll find someone who organised the Melbourne Cup suddenly has difficulty with organising what to take to the shower.
—Deb England, counsellor

For others, the disease strikes during retirement. John Silk was enjoying playing golf with his mates and spending time with his wife of 47 years when he was diagnosed in 2002. He was 66. It became obvious he needed to see a doctor after he fell backward as he cheered on the Wallabies at Olympic Stadium in 2002. He had a brain scan the following week, and soon after his neurologist delivered his diagnosis. 'The doctor saw me walk down the hall and said, "You've got Parkinson's." It was as quick as that.'

John was relatively calm at the time, compared with when he had been diagnosed with diabetes in 1987. He took that news harder because of the thought of using needles.

The neurologist put John on Parkinson's medication straight-away to relieve his symptoms. Before then, John couldn't write or shave properly, his movement was slow, and he was prone to freezing. He didn't experience any tremors when he was diagnosed.

Melbourne resident Nerissa Mapes was only 28 years old when she was diagnosed. She went to her GP to get a mole removed and mentioned problems with her left arm. She thought it was the result of a netball injury several years before. Her GP said it was nerve damage, but referred Nerissa to a neurologist just in case.

After having a series of MRI scans and blood tests, her diagnosis was made clear. But she wasn't happy with the way her neurologist delivered the news. 'He said, "As I told you last time, you've got Parkinson's." But he never mentioned it before, and I was on my own when he broke the news.'

Before being treated, Nerissa took an hour longer to get ready in the mornings. One day she was out with her parents at a restaurant and struggled with her meal. What was supposed to be an enjoyable evening out with her family reduced her to tears.

Nerissa's grandmother had the disease for more than a decade before she died in 2009.

> *My grandmother was bed-ridden in a nursing home and couldn't feed herself. She couldn't walk and barely spoke. That was my point of reference when I was diagnosed. I was kind of lucky enough to be rational and say that everyone's journey is different.*
> —Nerissa Mapes, diagnosed with Parkinson's in her 20s

Because Nerissa was so young when she was diagnosed, doctors carried out DNA testing, but they ruled out a genetic link. 'It's not hereditary or it wasn't linked to my grandmother. It's just the luck of the draw really,' Nerissa says.

Paula Argy's story

I guess when I think back, the first time my symptoms really became noticeable was on my wedding day. At the tender young age of 23, in front of a crowded church of 350 family and friends,

I was walking down the aisle holding a bouquet of my favourite flowers, tulips. My hands were trembling so much it looked like my bouquet was motorised! I put it down to a bad case of the jitters from emotions associated with my big day. Little did I know what was to transpire from my bouquet of 'shaky' tulips.

New symptoms began to appear over the next few years, which were really unsettling and would shake my world. I began to experience an overwhelming feeling of fatigue, particularly in the evening. I would lose my balance and stumble all over the place. My hands and feet would become rigid and my toes would clench and curl over. The symptoms seemed to be noticeably worse when I was tired, anxious or stressed. I was trying to juggle my career and the demands of working in the high-flying world of advertising with keeping house. I took care of all the domestic duties around the house. I loved to entertain so when I wasn't working I was planning elaborate dinner parties for my friends and family. Not knowing what was wrong with me was making things a lot worse. I was becoming very self-conscious, depressed and anxious about the symptoms and how I appeared to look to others. I would avoid social events, which was very difficult, as christenings, weddings and birthday parties were a weekly event in our family.

My concerns about the tremor were dismissed and misdiagnosed by many health professionals. At the age of 25, I went to see a neurologist and, after an MRI scan, was told that it was nothing, just a benign essential tremor. The neurologist prescribed medication, which had no noticeable effect on me. A family friend suggested I go down the naturopathic path. I went on liver detox diets, liver cleansing, and took copious amounts of vitamins, B6 and magnesium injections. After six months of treatment and bucket loads of money, my condition did not improve. The naturopath finally admitted defeat and referred me yet again to another neurologist.

On 12 May 1997, at the age of 27, I went to see another

specialist. I took my sister to the appointment, somehow knowing the news he was to give me wasn't going to be good. The neurologist said he knew exactly what was wrong with me and said he believed I had an extremely rare neurological condition in the family of Parkinson's and started me on Levodopa medication immediately. My sister and I just sat there stunned and in tears.

Once I commenced the Parkinson's medication my symptoms improved. That itself was a diagnosis. What followed the next few years was a series of tests, some involving hospitalisation, lumbar puncture testing of spinal fluid, nuclear brain scans where I was injected with radioactive dye and a brain scan was performed, and genetic blood tests, just to name a few.

I was devastated. What was to happen to me, to my dreams of having children? I was so young. I had goals and aspirations. I went off in a daze, not knowing what this really meant. I embarked on a mission to research this condition. I searched on the net and sought out information from the library, searching for the answers ... Parkinson's disease is a degenerative neurological condition and there is no known cause, prevention or cure. Not yet anyway!

John Ball's story

Every time I went out for a run my left foot would cramp up. I was 28 years old and couldn't run a kilometre without this absurd muscle cramping. That was my first signal of an approaching problem. As time wore on, the other signs appeared—difficulty standing up straight, getting stuck in places, knees and elbows that were stiff and sore, joints that ratcheted like worn old gears. I went to the doctors again and again, and they all shook their wise heads and said, 'Well, if I didn't know better, I'd say it looks a little like Parkinson's, but it can't be that. You're way too young. Way too healthy.'

The first one said: 'I think what you've got is choreoathetosis.' Well, it wasn't that, whatever that is.

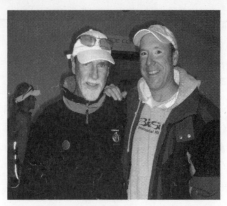

John (left) with a friend

The second one said: 'No, I think it's a circulation problem. Let's put you on a treadmill and wire you up with sensors.' Well, it wasn't that either.

The third chimed in: 'How about a brain tumour? That's always fun.' The CAT scans showed nothing abnormal.

Finally the mechanic in the group, the orthopaedic surgeon, said: 'Maybe it's just a mechanical problem. I think you've got the piriformis muscle pinching your sciatic nerve.' You know, he was so compelling I let him operate on my derriere, but the best I can say is that I eventually recovered from the surgery. In every case, the cramp always came back.

This sort of treatment went on for 12 years, until finally, the neurologist gave me a small packet of yellow tablets and told me to take one to see what effect it might have. I took the tablet just before a softball game. Our team was a bunch of guys from work, and I had been part of the team for five or six years. They had carried me as my ability declined from the outfielder to second baseman, from second base to pitcher, from pitcher to catcher. It got to the point where I couldn't throw the ball back to the pitcher without bouncing it. I couldn't throw a softball 15 metres. If I had to bat and actually hit the ball, they had to send a pinch runner to first base. But on the night I took that first yellow tablet, something magical happened.

By the third inning I was feeling better and into the game. Right there in the middle of the inning, our pitcher, Larry, came down from the mound and asked: 'What's going on John? You're standing up straight and throwing me the ball like the old days without bouncing it.'

'It must be these magic beans,' I said and showed him my oval-shaped yellow tablets.

I went home that night and looked up those tablets in my drug encyclopedia. It was a combination of levodopa and carbidopa called Sinemet 25/100. After 12 years of CAT scans and spinal taps, blood samples and even major surgery, there it was in simple print: 'For the treatment of Parkinson's disease'.

— Extract from John Ball's speech to the Parkinson's Congress in Sydney, 2008. He is the author of *Living Well and Running Hard: Lessons Learned from Living with Parkinson's Disease*

Other complications

As the disease progresses, people will experience complications that can be addressed with help from a neurologist or allied health professional.[24] Many of these complications are discussed in more detail in the following chapters. In many instances, these later complications do not respond to the main medications used to treat the movement problems of Parkinson's disease. Instead, other medication or strategies might help.

Difficulty with swallowing and chewing

The muscles used in swallowing can become rigid, slow and difficult to move in the later stages of the disease. This causes problems with swallowing food, drinks, saliva and medications, which can lead to chest infections and dehydration, and may make it difficult to get adequate nutrition. Early review by a speech pathologist is important if you experience these problems to reduce the risk of chest infections. Dietitians and occupational therapists can also help.

Communication changes

About half of all Parkinson's patients have problems with communicating because of the nature of the disease. They may speak too softly, hesitate before speaking, slur their words or speak too fast. At times people will struggle to take part in conversations, where that was not a problem before. A speech pathologist can teach strategies that may be very effective in helping to deal with these issues.

Urinary problems or constipation

As people with Parkinson's disease are often elderly, they can experience a range of problems that may interfere with the functioning of their bladder and bowel. At times the prostate is blamed for bladder and bowel changes, when Parkinson's disease itself may be the main culprit. In some patients, bladder and bowel problems can be the result of improper functioning of the autonomic nervous system. This system helps control the involuntary muscles and bodily functions that are not consciously directed. For example, the autonomic nervous system is responsible for regular heartbeats, intestinal movements and sweating.[25] In Parkinson's, some people may become incontinent, while others have trouble urinating. Constipation can also occur because the intestinal tract operates more slowly. Inactivity, a poor diet, or drinking too little fluid are also contributing factors. The presence of urinary problems may cause people to drink less fluid, which will worsen constipation. The medications used to treat Parkinson's disease can also make the problem worse. Adequate fluid, dietary fibre and exercise are important early lifestyle changes to keep bowels working.

Sexual dysfunction

Parkinson's disease often causes erectile dysfunction because it affects nerve signals from the brain, or because of poor blood circulation. Tremors or slowness of movement may also interfere with sexual function. This can be avoided by timing sex with good movement periods. Parkinson's-related depression or the use of some types of antidepressant medication can also lower sex drive. These problems are often treatable. In some cases, people become hypersexual (over-active) because of the dopamine agonist medications used to treat symptoms.

Skin problems

In Parkinson's disease, it is common for facial skin to become very oily, particularly on the forehead and around the nose, occasionally associated with reddening and pain (seborrheic dermatitis). The scalp may also become oily, resulting in dandruff. In other cases, the skin can become very dry. These problems are also the result of a poorly functioning autonomic nervous system. Standard treatments for skin problems can help. Excessive sweating, another common symptom, is usually controlled with medications used for Parkinson's disease.

Sleep problems

Patients might have difficulty maintaining good sleep patterns because of restlessness, nightmares and emotional dreams. Medications can also cause drowsiness or sudden onset of sleep during the day, upsetting normal sleep patterns. People who have Parkinson's disease should never take over-the-counter sleep aids without consulting their doctor. Vivid dreams may occasionally disrupt sleep and cause a person to hit out, risking injury to themselves or their partner. Treatments for these problems are often available and they can prove very effective.

2. Accepting the Diagnosis

I opted for denial, which in my case meant even more work. And when I wasn't on the job, I was drinking. At a time when I needed to draw my family closer, I shut them out. I feared that PD would keep me from being the father and husband I had promised to be.[1]

—Michael J. Fox, actor

Accepting a diagnosis of Parkinson's disease is easier said than done. Many people go through different emotional stages before accepting the diagnosis and taking control of their future. It's difficult for someone to embrace a future that is likely to rob them of their mobility and independence, and people absorb the shock of their diagnosis in different ways.

Parkinson's counsellor Deb England says younger people are often sent into a tailspin because they don't know what's going to happen next, whereas someone in their 70s might be more philosophical about their diagnosis and able to accept it more readily. Occupational therapist Dr Anne Hillman agrees older people may adapt to the illness more easily if, through life experience, they have developed lower expectations of their capabilities. 'It's not just specific to Parkinson's disease. Older people may have more strategies to adapt if they have already experienced changes that involve a decline in what they are able to do on a daily basis,' she says. 'Whereas younger people expect to increase or maintain their physical capacity.'

Because Brian has experienced many illnesses throughout our marriage, I wasn't that worried. I've seen his mum go through PD, but we now realise he's a lot worse than his mum ever was. I sort of knew what I was in for, so it wasn't as big a shock for me as it is for a lot of others.

—Pauline England, aged 73, wife and carer of a Parkinson's disease patient

Nerissa Mapes, aged 33, says she worries about what her future holds. 'I feel like my future is a bit of a question mark. I don't do much planning or thinking ahead. Having children is a pretty scary thing. I really want to have children, but fine motor skills are really important when you have a small baby. So that's a bit scary.' To cope with her fears, Nerissa has made a conscious decision to live in the now and keep healthy.

There are different types and degrees of acceptance. People might say 'well I still hate it [Parkinson's disease], but I accept that I've got this'.

—Dr Chris Basten, clinical psychologist

It's not unusual for people to go through stages of denial and anger, almost as if they are grieving over a loved one. They can also experience feelings of shock, anxiety and resentment. Clinical psychologist Dr Chris Basten says the 'why me?' question is a common one because patients feel like they've been dealt a cruel injustice. People find different ways of coping with anger and resentment. Some find comfort in religion or by becoming more introspective.

You can either stay home and wallow in it or try and make a difference. The best thing I did was talk to students because they need to understand the condition.

—Karen Rowland, diagnosed with Parkinson's in her 40s

It's a bit like death, in a sense. You become stunned and go through the grieving process. There's denial, anger and finally acceptance. Once you've reached acceptance it becomes a part of your life. The quicker you get your head around the fact that the disease isn't going to go away the better quality of life you'll have. Positive thinking is so important.

—Paula Argy, young mother with Parkinson's disease

Starting a family: Paula Argy's journey

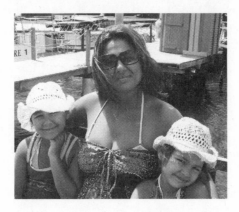

I began my ten-year-long journey of denial, grief, anger and then what I have come to know now as acceptance. I was not going to let this diagnosis beat me. There was no giving in to the illness or letting it dictate the terms of my life. I guess you could say I had youth and steadfast determination on my side. My quest and aspiration was to have children. I longed to be a mother.

I had left the stressful world of advertising, followed by a job in marketing and film distribution, and was now working for local government. At this point of my life, I was going through the stage of denial, thinking if I ignored my condition it would go away. My employer was unaware of my illness and I tried very hard to hide the symptoms. My husband and I spent the summer travelling around

Europe, which was quite physically and mentally exhausting. But I was so grateful that I had the opportunity to experience it.

I had my first child at age 30. It was an extremely difficult period of my life as I had to stay off the Parkinson's medication to ensure no harm came to my unborn baby. Not taking the medication meant that my symptoms came back in their fullest ferocity. My mobility was compromised. Walking, housework, driving became extremely difficult, let alone working. I took early maternity leave, which I told the company was due to complications in pregnancy. I could not let work see me this way. With the support of my loving family, nine months came and went and our first daughter Greta was born. My sole purpose and existence in this life was evident. I was so relieved that she was healthy and I was besotted straight away … my beautiful baby girl!

My battle of the mind, body and spirit was to continue. I went back on my medication, and then off again after two years when I became pregnant with our second child. The second pregnancy was definitely even more difficult than the first. This time I had an active toddler to chase after and chasing in my condition was a challenging feat! Another nine months of being housebound unable to move and again with the support of my family, my second gorgeous girl Mary was born. I just cried and cried the moment she was born, so relieved that she was okay and that I survived it all.

The few years that followed were extremely difficult. Two young children, our own business, a mortgage, a progressive illness and fears of what the future held for me and my young family. It was not easy. I fought it every day, just wanting the illness to go away. I felt guilty for being sick, even though logically I realised it was not my fault. I did not want to burden my family. I was falling deeper and deeper into a hole of blackness. The stress of it all took a toll on my health when I developed pneumonia and was hospitalised. It was then I sought help from the counselling service of Parkinson's NSW. I began the process of acceptance. I had gone through denial, fear and anger, and now I needed to accept.

Coping with Parkinson's

Feelings of anxiety often arise because people with Parkinson's fear they will lose control of their physical symptoms. Counsellor Deb England says people are worried about unwanted attention: 'What if I go out somewhere and I spill something? What if my shaking makes me obvious? What if I freeze or fall?'

Deb worked through those problems with a man who was fairly advanced in his Parkinson's and had trouble with mobility and speech. His daughter was getting married, and she wanted him to walk her down the aisle. But, as her wedding day approached, his anxiety levels increased. So Deb talked about his fears and drew up a 'worse-case scenario' plan, which he could manage. What would happen if he fell while walking her down the aisle? He was familiar with the church and knew there would be plenty of people to help in the event of a fall. But what would he say? They agreed on using humour to address a problem situation. He thought up a party line if he fell in the church: 'I suppose you thought I'd started at the reception.' Needless to say, there was no stumble. His pride was kept intact, and the wedding went without a hitch.

Then there are voice projection problems. People affected by speech difficulties are constantly asked to repeat themselves. At an event like a wedding, when there's a lot of competing noise, it may be very difficult for someone to make themselves understood, which can lead to some social anxiety. The lack of intonation or the inability to make gestures or eye contact makes patients worry that people will think they're not interested in what they have to say.

People who have communication problems often feel isolated because their speech is slow and they can't express their emotions very well. Some people also have trouble going to the toilet, so they're reluctant to leave the home. Others are embarrassed by their physical symptoms. Those feelings are often exacerbated by people's reactions.

Paula Argy says she'll often get strange looks from people when she's out walking. Parents at her children's pre-school didn't know she had the condition, and some assumed she was drunk when she walked through the playground. She believes that lack of awareness can make matters worse for people with Parkinson's.

Counsellor Deb England agrees, and says the only way to address the social stigma is to be open about the diagnosis so others don't make assumptions. 'For example, if you're having trouble getting money out of your wallet, then explain to the cashier that Parkinson's disease has affected you that day. That makes it easier for you to control the information without people making assumptions. If your gait is unsteady and you say it's because of Parkinson's, then people won't assume you're drunk.'

Deb England encourages people to disclose their condition to help others understand. But people should not feel they have to tell the world if they are normally a private person and are not so concerned about what others think.

> *Once people understand, they're more tolerant because*
> *Parkinson's disease changes every day. Some days you can*
> *do things and other days you can't. Your friends might not*
> *understand why.*
> —Karen Rowland, diagnosed with Parkinson's in her 40s

The lives of Parkinson's patients are ruled by their medication regime. Deb England says that when someone's medication has worn off, it's like their car has run out of petrol. Patients are terrified of being in a position where their medication starts to wear off.

'There is a lot of anxiety surrounding the condition,' she says. 'If that's not addressed or strategies aren't put in place, it will feed into depression.'

People often feel like they're losing control over their abilities, and focus on this during the course of the illness. It's important for people with Parkinson's to keep positive and find ways of adjusting.

> *People need to be able to accept, to learn and to live their*
> *life from day one and enjoy it. It doesn't matter what stage*
> *of Parkinson's they've got, they need to enjoy the day.*
> *Acceptance helps them get through the process of denial and*
> *to adjust using different approaches.*
> —Margarita Makoutonina, occupational therapist

> *The aim is to live well with Parkinson's. You don't want your*
> *identity characterised by the disease. It's a matter of accepting*
> *you have the condition and learning how to live well with it.*
> —Professor Meg Morris, physiotherapist

Occupational therapist Dr Anne Hillman agrees that a key to coping with the illness is to adapt to it. In her observations and studies, she has found people with Parkinson's disease struggle with their new identity. 'The idea that they are someone with a disease which has a label is quite difficult. It means they have to think hard about who they are and they need to redefine themselves to accommodate the fact they now have a disease.'

She says people may maintain their sense of self by modifying what they do without relinquishing it. For example, in a study she conducted, one woman with Parkinson's disease who has a large family was used to cooking lunch for up to ten people every Sunday. She was having trouble remembering recipes and managing her Sunday routine. So instead of cooking for a large group, she decided to keep the numbers small and cook more simply. She started inviting only a few people around for lunch at a time. This strategy worked well, and it meant she could maintain her role as the family matriarch.

Dr Hillman says persistence is an important weapon in dealing with daily challenges. 'People in my study told me they found that although something may not work today, it could work tomorrow.' Persistence in problem solving can help someone maintain a sense of control: 'Being flexible and trying out different strategies to deal with specific problems can provide good outcomes.' On the other hand, she found that if someone had to give up something that was really important to them, they sometimes did a psychological shuffle, convincing themselves that although it used to be important, it didn't matter to them so much now. They changed their expectations of themselves.

Conquering the black moods

You can't be positive all the time. I have my down days. If you have 20 good days and one bad, then enjoy the days that are good. You can't help getting depressed now and then, it's just a matter of how far it gets you.'
—John Silk, diagnosed with Parkinson's in his 60s

Depression affects nearly half of all Parkinson's patients and the biological reasons can't be ignored. Research suggests that depression takes hold because the production of neurotransmitters that affect mood (such as serotonin) is impaired. So there are biological processes at play that can lead to someone developing depression. There are also psychological challenges that come with the compromised motor control and social isolation of the disease. Mood can vary considerably during the day in conjunction with movement or medication cycles. While this is not strictly labelled depression, which is by definition a fixed and longer lasting mood disorder, these mood fluctuations can be very disabling. They may also respond to changes in medication and other interventions used for depression.

Features of Parkinson's disease, such as apathy and slow movement, can be easily confused with depression. So what should someone look out for?

The symptoms of depression include:[2]

- an uncharacteristic, lengthy, period of sadness
- loss of interest in regular activities
- feeling worthless
- tiredness
- disturbed sleep
- changes in appetite
- negative thoughts and feelings.

Medication

Moderate to severe forms of depression are usually treated with medication, especially if people experience symptoms for more than two weeks. Antidepressants usually take one to three weeks to work effectively, and they should not be started or stopped without medical advice, as side effects can occur. Some of the newer antidepressants can worsen the symptoms of Parkinson's in some people (see the contraindications chart, pages 185–90). Professor Malcolm Horne says neurologists prefer to prescribe some of the older drugs, such as Endep (which belongs to a class of drug called tricyclic antidepressants).

A recent study by the University of South Australia found tricyclic antidepressants were more effective than selective serotonin reuptake inhibitors to treat people with Parkinson's disease.[3] Selective serotonin reuptake inhibitors, such as Zoloft and Prozac, are the most commonly prescribed antidepressants in Australia, and are often less sedating than the older antidepressants such as Endep.

People who experience only mild or moderate forms of depression may find psychological treatments, such as cognitive behaviour therapy, helpful. This therapy enables people to address negative feelings by using practical self-help strategies. For example, if someone is depressed and feels powerless to change in any way, then a therapist would help the patient to identify these false and unhealthy thoughts and work out ways to avoid them.[4] Interpersonal therapy helps people to improve their relationships so they can feel better.

'The medication has a certain level of effectiveness but it doesn't help everybody. The main thing that helps depression is exercise and maintaining good social relationships,' says psychologist Dr Chris Basten.

Peter McWilliam says he was shocked when he found out he was suffering depression. His specialist picked up the signs and he was prescribed antidepressants for a few months. Peter believed this fixed a quarter of his symptoms. 'It can manifest not only in being miserable and down, but physically. You lack drive and it can slow you down physically, which is what happened to me.'

John Ball: A patient's perspective

For most people, Parkinson's is a very isolating disease. It's like a net thrown over us. That net restrains us and shrinks our world into smaller and smaller circles of contact with the world. It is this continual sense of loss that is so depressing for many Parkinson's patients: loss of skills, mobility, jobs and friendships. With this continual loss comes a sense of diminished value, of losing not only your abilities, but also your sense of worth in the world. Attached to that loss is a sense of guilt; you live with the knowledge that what Parkinson's disease takes from you, you no longer have available to give to those you love. My friend Dan is in his early forties and has had Parkinson's for nearly ten years. He is also a new father. His tremors are occasionally severe enough to make him reluctant to hold his baby daughter Lucy in his hands, because he's afraid he'll drop her. He's concerned that she will think him a cold and distant father rather than a vital part of her life. How will this play out over the next 20 years as she grows up?

— Extract from speech to 2008 Parkinson's Congress, Sydney

The importance of exercise

There is some evidence that exercise may also help alleviate depression, although it's not known which form of exercise is best. Beyondblue, a national group that provides information to sufferers and carers, says exercise can help to improve sleep patterns, increase perceived coping ability and block negative thoughts that make depression worse.

Jogging, weightlifting, walking, stationary cycling and weight training have all been found to help prevent or treat mild to moderate depression. For people with Parkinson's, the type of activity chosen will depend on the stage of the illness and whether the exercise is compatible with their motor and cognitive skills.

Other strategies for managing depression

While complementary treatments may offer relief for people with depression, generally, this approach might not be the ideal solution for those with Parkinson's disease.[5] Professor Malcolm Horne says it's not clear that people with Parkinson's disease will benefit from these strategies. 'There is a greater than expected incidence of depression in people with PD and there are reasonably good grounds to suspect that it is more likely to be a neurochemical problem, and so medical solutions will be necessary.' Nevertheless, some people believe alternative therapies are worth a try. Some of those options are listed below.[6]

Acupuncture
A review of eight studies found acupuncture reduced symptoms of depression. Western medicine believes acupuncture may

stimulate nerves, which results in the release of serotonin and norepinephrine. Serotonin is a chemical in the brain that influences a person's mood, while norepinephrine is a hormone and neurotransmitter which is released during stressful situations, similar to adrenaline.

Fish oil supplements

Omega-3 fatty acids are found in certain fish, plants and nut oil. Omega-3 supplements appear to work as a treatment for depression, but the evidence is small.

Massage

There can be short-term improvement in mood after one massage, and long-term benefits if regular massages are received over several days or weeks.

Relaxation training

Stress management techniques may be used as a treatment for anxiety. They appear to work, but do not appear to be as effective as psychological therapies, as the benefit tends to be short lived; although, with regular practice the benefit can be longer lasting.

St John's wort supplements

A traditional herbal remedy for depression, St John's wort appears to be helpful in mild cases, and when taken alone has fewer side effects than antidepressants. But the supplement interacts with many medications, affecting the way they work, which can produce serious side effects. Patients thinking of trying St John's wort to treat their depression should get expert advice. You should also mention to the doctor that you are taking alternative medications, as they are frequently omitted from formal lists of therapy and may interact with new medication.

Yoga
This is a promising treatment for depression as it reduces stress and improves relaxation. More research is needed on the benefits of yoga as a treatment.

Depression questionnaire

People diagnosed with Parkinson's disease who feel they may be developing depression can use the questionnaire on the following page, which was designed to help measure depression in the medically ill. It does not include symptoms, such as fatigue, sleep or appetite disturbance and weight change, that are common to both depression and many illnesses.

The measure only includes mental processes because the aim is to reflect the quintessential mood state of depression. The questionnaire was tested in general practitioner populations and its use as a screening measure for depression has been established. The scale excludes items on suicidal ideation and plans. These should be addressed during a face-to-face interview with a clinician.

Instructions
Consider the following questions and rate how true each one is in relation to how you have been feeling lately (in the last two to three days) compared with how you usually or normally feel. Tick the most relevant option: Not True/Slightly True/ Moderately True/Very True.

Scoring the questionnaire
Allocate 0 points for each Not True answer; 1 point each for Slightly True; 2 points each for Moderately True; and 3 points each for Very True.

A total score of 9 or more suggests probable or definite depression.

	Not true	Slightly true	Moderately true	Very true
1. Are you stewing over things?				
2. Do you feel more vulnerable than usual?				
3. Are you being self-critical and hard on yourself?				
4. Are you feeling guilty about things in your life?				
5. Do you find that nothing seems to be able to cheer you up?				
6. Do you feel as if you have lost your core and essence?				
7. Are you feeling depressed?				
8. Do you feel less worthwhile?				
9. Do you feel hopeless or helpless?				
10. Do you feel more distant from other people?				

Reprinted with permission of the Black Dog Institute[7]

Where to go for help

Your treating neurologist or GP should be the first port of call when seeking help for depression. They may want to refer you to a psychologist or psychiatrist. Psychiatrists are doctors who make medical assessments and prescribe medication. Psychologists, social workers and occupational therapists in mental health all focus on providing non-medical treatment for depression. The Australian Psychological Society website is at www.psychology.org.au and is a helpful resource when looking for specialist help.

A Medicare rebate can be claimed for psychological treatments when a patient is referred to a psychologist, social worker or occupational therapist by their treating general practitioner.

Useful addresses

Beyondblue: the national depression initiative
    www.beyondblue.org.au
    1300 22 4636

Black Dog Institute
    www.blackdoginstitute.org.au
    (02) 9382 4523

Carers Australia
    www.carersaustralia.com.au
    1800 242 636

Parkinson's Australia
    www.parkinsons.org.au
    1800 644 189

3. Taking Charge of Your Health

A team of experts can help people with Parkinson's, their families and carers to accept the diagnosis, help with disability and manage movement and cognitive disturbance when their medications fail.

—Margarita Makoutonina, Victorian Comprehensive Parkinson Program

Because Parkinson's disease is such a complex illness, it needs to be managed by a diverse group of experts who can monitor each symptom as the illness develops. Each patient's experience is different, which means advice that is tailored to the individual is particularly important.

The rights of people who have Parkinson's disease are outlined in a charter that was drawn up in 1997 by the European Parkinson's Disease Association and the World Health Organization.

The charter states patients have the right to:

- be referred to a doctor with a special interest in Parkinson's disease
- receive an accurate diagnosis
- have access to support services
- receive continuous care
- take part in managing their illness.

The best starting point for a patient is finding the right neurologist, particularly one who has an interest in Parkinson's disease or, better still, someone who has carried out research in the field.

The team approach

Melbourne neurologist Professor Robert Iansek believes a team approach is the best way of managing Parkinson's disease. He says the disease is a complex illness and movement problems are just the tip of the iceberg. It can also affect thinking, behaviour and mood. Because Parkinson's disease cannot be cured, these problems get worse over time. Professor Iansek has used more than 25 years of research knowledge to develop a specific multidisciplinary rehabilitation program for people with the illness.

Team approach to managing Parkinson's

Professor Iansek's treatment team includes:

- doctors (GP, neurologist, neurosurgeon)
- physiotherapists
- occupational therapists
- psychologists and psychiatrists
- social workers
- speech pathologists
- dietitians
- nurses.

The comprehensive multidisciplinary program, which started 16 years ago, uses the skills of doctors and allied health professionals to ensure patients are not only treated for their symptoms but are able to learn strategies to cope with daily living. The program looks after 5000 patients in Victoria. Professor Iansek says:

You need to have experts in all of these areas ... to deal with the complexities of the disease. Medications aren't always the be all and end all. It's sometimes difficult to keep people on an even keel so we provide them with a back-up system that enables them to function normally.

When simple tasks become more challenging, this back-up system teaches patients and carers strategies so they can go about their daily life with much more ease and confidence. Patients are taught how to get out of bed, how to avoid getting stuck in doorways and how to cope with everyday activities such as showering and dressing.

The Victorian Comprehensive Parkinson Program is run through public and private hospitals, five multidisciplinary clinics and 20 inpatient beds, as well as outreach and carer support services. It is the only centre of excellence in Australia, as defined by the National Parkinson's Foundation in the United States, and one of just 43 medical centres in the world forming a network that delivers a comprehensive program to address all symptoms of the disease.

Unless people with Parkinson's have a program to cater to their particular needs ... they're left on their own. They're left to fend for themselves.

—Professor Robert Iansek

We're not here to tell you what to do, we're here to support you. As the disease progresses, many people are left to manage on their own. They get medical help, but they're not getting anything else. It's the other support that people really need.

—Dr Anne Hillman, Sydney occupational therapist

Continuity of care is also important for patients so that their symptoms can be closely monitored over the course of their illness and treatment strategies are shaped accordingly. Professor Iansek says:

> We're probably the only program that provides inpatient management. People with middle-stage or advanced Parkinson's disease need to be admitted to hospital and monitored so their medication can be adjusted to their particular needs because everyone is so different.

Skilled nurses monitor patients every hour to fine-tune the dose and timing intervals for medication. Most people are in hospital for a few weeks while their medication is adjusted, and rehabilitation training is provided. 'You can achieve tremendous improvements in medication with this sort of approach.' says Professor Iansek, who believes there are not enough team-based programs available to patients in Australia:

> People think [a team-based program] is expensive to set up but it's not. Most delivery models in Australia are reactive. Our program is very proactive and preventative in the sense you identify issues and deal with them before they become major. It's the way people with Parkinson's want to be treated.

Sydney's Concord Hospital and Perth's Osborne Park Hospital also provide multidisciplinary care.

A patient's perspective

Peter McWilliam, aged 67, who was diagnosed nearly two decades ago, says that anyone with a chronic illness will say our medical system is never good enough.

> Our support groups work very well. It's the funding for medical services that's lacking. In Britain, they have nurse specialists who are highly trained and can take over a lot

of the load neurologists carry. We need a good network of clinical nurses in Australia, among other things, like respite care, which is inadequate.

Medications

Australia has one third less treatment options than Europe or North America.

—HTA, *Help for Today: Hope for Tomorrow*

Many people with Parkinson's disease miss out on newer treatments because they are deemed too expensive and are not subsidised under the Australian Pharmaceutical Benefits Scheme (PBS). Sydney neurologist Dr Victor Fung says the PBS has very strict criteria for proving the cost benefit of any medication. That makes it tough for many patients, whose disease comes on late in their working life and causes slow and gradual impairment without causing death or the need for high-level care at an early stage. 'That means many of the costs are borne silently by the patient and their carer and family.'

Due to the interaction of many medications with Parkinson's therapy, or because of the condition itself, traditional medications supported by the PBS may not be helpful or can cause significant side effects. Central Coast neurologist Associate Professor Scott Whyte says that the relatively small number of people with Parkinson's disease who need these specific medications has meant that the PBS has continued to neglect supporting many of these vital and available medications in Parkinson's disease, at the same time as supporting them in other conditions.

Nevertheless, a range of medications are available to treat the disease, and drugs continue to be the main form of treatment for people with Parkinson's.

The preferred medication is levodopa (L-dopa), a drug that is very effective in controlling movement problems but it doesn't stop the disease from progressing.

Levodopa

Levodopa is a naturally occurring amino acid which, once absorbed by the brain, is converted to dopamine. However, a large proportion of levodopa is transformed into dopamine in tissue outside the brain, which can cause side effects, such as vomiting and low blood pressure. To prevent these side effects, levodopa is combined with carbidopa or benserazide.[1]

Medication names, and forms
The most common names for levodopa drugs are:

- Sinemet (levodopa + carbidopa)
- Kinson (levodopa + carbidopa)
- Madopar (levodopa + benserazide).

These medications may be found as standard tablets or capsules, and in rapid-release tablets and as slow-release preparations (these preparations are the same as the standard tablet form).

Side effects
Side effects may include nausea, increased dreaming, dizziness and, in the long term, hallucinations and dyskinesias (involuntary movements).[2]

PBS
All levodopa-class drugs are subsidised by the government under the Pharmaceutical Benefits Scheme.

Long-term use
After several years on levodopa medication, patients may begin

to deteriorate and experience fluctuations in their mobility. This is called the 'on' and 'off' effect, indicating when the drug is apparently working and when it is not. Doctors say response to the drug becomes more complicated and erratic.

The classic consensus is that about 50 per cent of patients develop motor fluctuations after five years of levodopa treatment. Recent studies have suggested that the frequency is even higher.

—*European Neurology*, March 2009

Neurologist Dr Michael Hayes says people with early Parkinson's disease become more dependent on the drug as their own reservoir of dopamine diminishes. 'As the L-dopa is broken down you get a peak dose and then over the new few hours it wears off. Dopamine per se is pretty effective. The way it's delivered becomes less effective for the patient.'

After long-term use of the drug, changes called plasticity occur within the brain. 'This means the drugs alter the way the brain responds to them. The brain can become supersensitive, causing unpredictable fluctuations,' says neurologist Dr Victor Fung. 'Sometimes problems like these can be overcome by increasing the dosage or by the patient taking smaller doses at more frequent intervals,' says neurologist Dr Scott Whyte.

Dr Whyte says that as time passes the L-dopa based medications may begin wearing off at a faster rate. People may be used to taking their medication at 'roughly' the correct time or when they begin to feel the therapy wearing off. However, the benefit starts to wear off sooner, resulting in unexpected freezing or those episodes may become more frequent. For these people, taking the medication within a few minutes of the designated time can be crucial. In that case, a timer is useful in reminding someone when to take their medication. For people who experience rapid wearing off, medication may need to be taken before the first symptoms of wearing off appear. At times a hospital visit is recommended so medication can be adjusted appropriately. However, Dr Whyte says simply taking the medication on time might produce enough benefits that changes won't be warranted.

When L-dopa based medications are first prescribed, it is commonly recommended that they be taken with food, or after eating. This is to reduce the risk of nausea and vomiting, which can occur when the medication is started. Over time the nausea settles and taking medication with food may benefit by slowing its absorption. Dr Whyte says: 'If the effects of the tablets appear to fail when taken with food or soon after a meal, then it's best to take the tablets half an hour before or one and a half hours after a meal. This may improve medication response. Like most things, if you're not experiencing any problems, then you won't need to change the way the medication is taken.'

In some cases, a low-protein diet may improve the absorption of the drug.[3] Dr Whyte warns that a dietitian should be consulted, as nutritional deficiencies may occur if the diet is not structured well.

What the patients say

Karen Rowland is in her 50s and has been on dopamine therapy for nine years. She needs to take her regular medications on time and avoids caffeine and protein within half an hour of taking levodopa. 'You can't have a cup of coffee or cheese sandwich when your medication is due,' she says. 'Everything revolves around your medication, which is annoying.'

Karen takes Madopar four times a day, Sifrol (dopamine agonist) three times a day, and a slow-release Sinemet at night so she doesn't wake up stiff in the mornings. The amount of medication has been gradually increased over time, and in the past year she has noticed periods when her symptoms are unpredictable and return during the day. This is known as the 'wearing off' effect.

> *When I do something that's hard, the dopamine wears out faster.*
>
> —Karen Rowland, diagnosed in her 40s

Peter McWilliam was diagnosed in 1992, at age 50. For 15 years, he took a cocktail of drugs, but as his disease progressed, he needed more medication, which caused him to experience dyskinesias: his arms and legs began to move involuntarily, and his face began to twist. Peter says:

> *It's pretty much like seeing someone with cerebral palsy. It's that sort of body movement. Levodopa was working erratically after a while. Some days it worked, other days not. When you're 'off' you're trembling and ultimately you can't move at all and that's pretty uncomfortable. The drug benefits begin to wear out. It was fairly frustrating. Luckily I'm a sedentary person. I like reading, but you can't hold your body still to read a book with dyskinesia.*

Peter finally resorted to deep brain stimulation, a surgical treatment for Parkinson's disease that is becoming more widely used. Since having his operation, Peter doesn't rely too heavily on his medications and the doses have been dramatically reduced.

John Silk, who is in his early 70s, says dyskinesias (involuntary movements) can be a terrible side-effect of taking medications for many years. He takes up to a dozen tablets a day to help him to function properly. John knows that he has to take his medication on time, or his symptoms will get the better of him. 'I've got a quarter of an hour window.

If I don't get them inside a quarter of an hour, I start to perspire, I can't move and it's not fun,' he says.

Nerissa Mapes, aged 33, says that her medications have become an important part of her life. She takes a dopamine agonist (described below), and was recently prescribed Madopar.

> *When I skip my medication, I know exactly how bad I can be. Things slow right down. When paying for groceries it takes forever. I don't freeze, but I find everything much, much harder.*
>
> —Nerissa Mapes, diagnosed in her 20s

Dopamine agonists

This group of drugs can be used with levodopa or taken alone. They mimic the action of dopamine in the brain. They are considered weaker agents than levodopa because they are less potent, but the drug tends to stay in the body for much longer.

Dopamine agonists are used in the treatment of early Parkinson's disease to avoid the need for levodopa, and they may delay or reduce the likelihood of developing dopa-induced involuntary movements. The agonist drugs also help to reduce motor fluctuations in later disease.[4]

Medication names

The most common names for agonist drugs are:

- Sifrol (pramipexole)
- Requip (ropinirole)
- Cabaser (cabergoline)
- Permax (pergolide mesylate)
- Parlodel (bromocriptine mesylate)
- Kripton (bromocriptine mesylate)
- Apomine (apomorphine hydrochloride).

Sifrol
Side effects

Drugs such as Sifrol are more likely to provoke hallucinations, confusion and psychosis than levodopa. Sifrol can also cause ankle swelling. Excessive drowsiness is more common than other agonist drugs and Sifrol can cause a sudden onset of sleep without warning. Patients who still drive need to be especially aware of this. Unlike other medications, there does not appear to be any increased risk of heart-valve damage.[5]

Agonist drugs have been shown to increase the risk of compulsive behaviour. Hypersexuality and excessive shopping, eating and medication use, and repetitive purposeless activities have been reported in patients taking dopamine agonists, especially in high doses.[6]

PBS

Sifrol is subsidised for patients who are also taking levodopa.

Drug Cost Me the Lot: Banker

Tom Leonard, New York

12 July 2008

A former Wall Street banker is suing the makers of a drug for Parkinson's Disease, blaming it for triggering a 'pathological' gambling addiction that cost him $3 million.

Randolph Simens, 55, said he took Mirapex (pramipexole) between 2002 and 2007 after suffering from hand tremors and being diagnosed with Parkinson's.

He said the drug 'put a little tickle in me and then snowballed within a month' as his previous occasional recreational gambling spiralled into all-night online gambling sessions, risky share investments and frequent trips to casinos.

Mr Simens, from Armonk, New York, said his biggest one-day loss came when $US400,000 was wiped off the value of shares he had rashly bought.

His gambling habit became so severe that he even plundered the bank accounts of his two children, a court was told.

'It ruined me. I became like a robot and I was just pissing away money,' he said.

'It's stupidity. I just couldn't stop.'

He has accused three international drug makers—Boehringer Ingelheim, Pfizer, and Pharmacia and Upjohn—of breach of warranty, negligence and negligent representation.

Mr Simens, who is suing for his losses, claims the companies failed to warn users of the possible side effects.

A link between the drugs and possible compulsive behaviour has been known for several years. In 2005, a US study found they could make patients addicted to gambling as well as boosting their appetite for sex, food and alcohol.

Mr Simens said he joined a gamblers' support group and within five weeks of getting off Mirapex had stopped gambling. 'I'm better, but I'm broke.'

According to his lawsuit, the defendants 'had a duty to provide adequate warnings and instruction for Mirapex, to use reasonable care to design a product that is not reasonably dangerous to users, and to adequately test their product'. Boehringer Ingelheim started noting on the drug's label in 2005 that there had been reports saying 'compulsive behaviours' could result from its use.

The company, which is facing similar suits around the country, denies there is scientific evidence proving the link to gambling. A spokesman said the company would vigorously defend the lawsuit. Pfizer said the company had not marketed Mirapex since 2005, adding that it had 'acted reasonably and appropriately' during the period it was involved with the drug.

—Courtesy *The Age*, Melbourne

Cabaser, Permax, Parlodel, Kripton

Side effects

These drugs are more likely to provoke hallucinations, confusion and psychosis than levodopa. This group of drugs can also cause swelling. They are not recommended for patients with unstable coronary heart disease or peripheral vascular disease.

Up to 3 per cent of patients develop thickening of tissue (fibrotic reactions) in organs such as the lungs which can affect their function, but Dr Victor Fung says these changes are reversible if they are detected early enough. Around 33 per cent of patients taking Permax (pergolide) develop heart valve fibrosis, which can cause heart valves to damage and leak, so regular monitoring is highly recommended.[7]

Cabaser (cabergoline) may also cause heart valve problems or may affect lung and kidney function. Tests are recommended before and during the taking of this drug to identify the presence of any underlying disease, which would be a reason for not prescribing the drug. Scans should be carried out every 6–18 months.

Cabergoline and pergolide carry black-box safety warnings on the packaging, and the drugs are being prescribed less by Australian neurologists because of concerns about potential complications.

PBS

All listed.

What the patients say

Nerissa Mapes, aged 33, says the agonist drug Cabaser induced strange behaviour, such as waking up in the middle of the night and wanting to do the ironing.

Karen Rowland, aged 56, says she became a compulsive shopper: 'I've bought 16 white hats, and given them away. If I'm walking past a shop and see a white hat, I still want to buy it, even though I don't need it.' Karen has also heard similar stories. 'One chap has got four pencil cases of gel pens. Another woman has bought so many toilet rolls she has stacked them in her shower.'

In Melbourne, a class action was announced in 2008 after several patients developed gambling disorders from the drugs Cabaser and Permax. Amanda Spillare of Parkinson's Victoria, told the ABC's *7.30 Report* that 'about 7 per cent of people on dopamine agonists will experience a problem with impulse control'.

Apomine (apomorphine hydrochloride)

Apomine is a very potent dopamine agonist and it's considered more powerful than other drugs in this class. Administration is only by injection under the skin, as either a single injection when needed or via a small infusion pump carried in a pouch. The pouch is connected to a thin tube and a fine needle is left under the skin during the infusion. The needle is removed daily and medication in the pump refilled. It is often prescribed for people who have advanced disease to help reduce the number and severity of freezing episodes and stiffness (or 'off' periods). It becomes effective within 5–10 minutes of injection and the effects last for about an hour as a single injection; or continuously throughout the day and/or night, if using an infusion pump.

Side effects

This drug can cause severe nausea and vomiting, which doctors treat by prescribing Motilium (taken beforehand). Nausea is nearly always managed with medication; after being on apomorphine for a short period of time the body gets used to the medication, and anti-nausea therapy is no longer required.

PBS

Apomine is listed for patients severely disabled by motor fluctuations who don't respond to other therapy.

Fay Mongan's story

Sydney resident Fay Mongan, aged 75, was told she had
Parkinson's disease in the mid-1990s after being misdiagnosed
several years before. She had been told her symptoms were the
result of a mini-stroke. In 1993, Fay's specialist was 90 per cent
certain she had Parkinson's disease so he prescribed levodopa,
which worked well. Fay was then prescribed the controversial
agonist Cabaser to give her more of a boost. Her doctor told her
to start on 1 milligram, but said that she should stop taking the
drug straightaway if she experienced any funny spells (episodes
of compulsive behaviour). Unlike many other people, Fay handled
the medication quite well and didn't suffer any side effects such
as problem gambling.

After a while, Fay failed to respond to her main medications,
including Madopar and Comtan. She began to struggle physically
and couldn't walk or move. Her husband Dan would have to
carry her when she needed to get from one place to another. She
had difficulty doing everyday things, including watering her many
pot plants. She couldn't continue with her favourite hobbies,
such as sewing or cooking. It became harder to concentrate and
picking up an iron or threading a needle was no longer possible.
Her neurologist thought it was better that she see someone
about starting another drug, called Apomine (apomorphine).

The drug is only available through hospital pharmacies. Fay
was told she would have to wait six months for the hospital to
supply the medication. At another hospital, doctors needed
clearance from the hospital drug committee to allow its use.
Finally, five months after making enquiries, Fay was booked
to have the injection. She was taken off all medications so
that doctors could assess how much Apomine she needed to
take. During the nine hours without medication, her symptoms
returned and she became a complete wreck. 'Her hands and
feet shook like mad and her eyes were almost closed. All I
wanted to do was cry,' says husband Dan. Nurses gave her a

small dose of Apomine, which was injected into her stomach. They then gave her another dose. Soon she was up, walking and clapping her hands. Everyone was amazed at how she was able to move. At home, she uses a pump that's attached to a belt around her waist, so the medication is given continuously throughout the day.

Dan says her turnaround has been remarkable. She can now do her favourite things again. Her grandchildren recently gave her a birthday card saying 'Nanna, we didn't think you'd be here.'

Fay gets the occasional bout of freezing, but nothing like she experienced before. The biggest problem remaining is her inability to sleep. Sometimes she'll get a good sleep, but most times though Fay will wake up to four times a night. Fay's hallucinations continue. Once she thought there were people at her bedside. Another time she saw her late mother-in-law standing at the wardrobe, waiting for her to wake up. Dan says so long as the episodes don't turn nasty, they can live with the hallucinations. Fay doesn't see monsters jumping out of the ceiling like she used to. The hallucinations are not as disturbing, and they happen only rarely. She has managed to get her life back, and that's what counts.

COMT (catechol-o-methyl transferase) inhibitors
These are taken in conjunction with levodopa and help make it more effective by preventing its breakdown in the gut and blood.

Medication names
The most common names for COMT inhibitors are:

- Stalevo (levodopa/carbidopa/entacapone—three drugs are in one tablet)
- Comtan (entacapone).

Side effects

Two common side effects are an increase in dyskinesia (involuntary movements) and diarrhoea. A harmless side effect is discoloured urine. Dyskinesia is often tackled by altering the dose or time the medication is given. Doctors say there isn't any effective way of treating diarrhoea.

PBS

Stalevo and Comtan are both listed.

Amantadine

This drug is an anti-viral agent that has anti-Parkinsonian effects. It is used to suppress dyskinesia and slightly reverses movement problems.

Medication name

- Symmetrel (amantadine hydrochloride).

Side effects

These are rare but can include insomnia, hallucinations, confusion and mottled rash on legs. There are no specific remedies for insomnia. If a patient experiences hallucinations, doctors would recommend stopping the drug or reducing other medications. No treatment is needed for leg rash.

PBS

Listed.

Anticholinergics

These drugs block the effect of acetylcholine, another chemical of the brain, so its levels can be balanced with dopamine. They are useful in treating tremor, particularly among younger patients. Drugs in this class are usually taken in conjunction with other medication as they only relieve tremor and stiffness, not other movement problems such as slowness of movement or dyskinesia. Their benefit for stiffness, however, is not as good as other medication.

Medication names
The most common names for these drugs are:

- Artane (benzhexol hydrochloride)
- Congentin (benztropine mesylate)
- Akineton (biperiden hydrochloride).

Side effects
Dry mouth, memory impairment, confusion, constipation, blurred vision, worsening of glaucoma (unrelated to Parkinson's) and urinary retention may all occur. About 30 to 50 per cent of people may experience some of these side effects. It's recommended that treatment be stopped if there are intolerable side effects. It may be difficult to come off these drugs after they have been used for a long time.[8]

PBS
All are listed.

Monoamine Oxidase Type B inhibitors
This group of drugs inhibit the enzyme responsible for the breakdown of dopamine in the brain. This helps to reduce motor fluctuations.

Medication names
The most common names for these drugs are:

- Selgene
- Eldepryl (selegiline hydrochloride).

Side effects

Nightmares, hallucinations and confusion, worsening of dyskinesia may all occur. This drug can also affect serotonin levels in the brain, which can improve mood slightly. Serious reactions may occur if patients are also given pethidine for serious pain relief or certain types of antidepressants.

PBS

Listed for late-stage disease.

New research

Another drug in this class of Monoamine Oxidase B inhibitors called Rasagiline (azilect) has been investigated by researchers in the United States. Dr C Warren Olanow from Mount Sinai School of Medicine told ABC America: 'It's the first time we've defined a drug that looks like it slows the rate of disease progression.' The 18-month study, involving 1176 patients with untreated, early-stage Parkinson's disease, was published in the *New England Journal of Medicine* in 2009. The report concluded: 'While early treatment with Rasagiline at a dose of 1mg per day provided daily benefits consistent with a possible disease-modifying effect, early treatment at a dose of 2mg did not. Because of the different outcomes, the results must be interpreted with caution.'[9] The drug is not yet available in Australia.

New medications and preparations

New preparations of L-dopa based medication are becoming available. One of these is a suspension of L-dopa (Duodopa), which is infused via a pump through a tube placed into the stomach. For people with severe movement problems this type of therapy is offering improved function over oral treatments.

Neupro (rotigotine)

This is the only skin patch available to treat symptoms of early Parkinson's disease. The patch allows the drug to be slowly absorbed through the skin into the bloodstream, helping to keep a consistent flow of the drug into the patient's system. The patch is replaced every 24 hours. The drug delivered by the patch is in the dopamine agonist class of drugs, and shares the benefit and side-effect profile of these drugs. It can be used on its own or in combination with other Parkinson's treatments.

Side effects

Most common side effects of using the patch include skin reactions, dizziness, vomiting, drowsiness and insomnia. As mentioned, the drug shares the side-effects of others in its class, which can include sudden onset of sleep, hallucinations and decreased blood pressure. Some patients may experience repetitive meaningless actions, excessive gambling and increased sex drive.

PBS

Not listed.

Duodopa (levodopa/carbidopa)

Duodopa is a new treatment for patients in the mid to late stages of the disease. It is similar to Sinemet, but is available in a gel form, which is delivered directly into the small bowel (using a tube passed though the stomach and a pump), allowing the medication to flow continuously. The constant flow achieves a more stable control of symptoms. Doctors say this is a highly effective treatment. Most patients have little trouble managing the pump and tubing, though a lot of education should be given beforehand. Only those patients comfortable with the requirements should undergo this treatment.

Side effects
Surgery is required to place the tube, which can result in complications. It is currently a very expensive treatment.

PBS
Not listed.

What the patients say.
Paula Argy, aged 39, says she's been asked to try Duodopa and Apomine to better control the fluctuations she experiences. But she's not ready to have treatments that involve injection or carrying a pump, which she believes would compromise her active lifestyle. 'I'm a pretty compliant patient but I feel I'm not there yet. I'm not mentally there yet. I've got kids and I'm young. I'm managing okay with existing medications.' She has learned to take her pills on time to prevent any problems. 'I have them on time, all through the day and all through the night. I'm quite bad when I'm off medication. I can't move. If I missed a tablet by half an hour, I would be "off". I wouldn't be able to walk or stand up.'

Drug interactions
Many patients require additional medication to address the side effects associated with taking Parkinson's drugs. There is a list of the drugs that may interfere with a patient's treatment or may worsen the symptoms of the disease on pages 185–90.

Useful addresses
- Pharmaceutical Benefits Scheme: www.pbs.gov.au (click on PBS for consumers to find out cost of drugs)
- National Prescribing Service: www.nps.org.au (for information on medications)
- Medicare Australia: www.medicareaustralia.gov.au (for

information on subsidies) click on individual & families, claims & cover.

Surgery
Deep brain stimulation (DBS)

Deep brain stimulation (DBS) is an option for patients who have taken standard medications for a number of years, but the drugs are either not lasting long enough or the patient has started to experience side effects. Some people assume DBS is a treatment of 'last resort', but Melbourne neurosurgeon Richard Bittar says that's not the case: 'It's offered by doctors when all other reasonable options have been tried, and have either failed or not been tolerated very well.'

This treatment can reduce the severity and duration of motor fluctuations. Sydney neurologist Dr Victor Fung says DBS is not better than medications when they're working at their peak, with two exceptions.

1. It can relieve tremor that is resistant to medication.
2. It can reduce dyskinesias (involuntary movements).

> *The medication (levodopa) was working erratically after a while. The drug benefits begin to wear out. Everyone said I was bad. ... so I decided to take the plunge.*
>
> —Peter McWilliam, on his decision to have
> deep brain stimulation

DBS is a surgical procedure that involves implanting an electrode or thin wire through the top of the skull into the area of the brain that causes the Parkinson's symptoms. The electrode is connected to an extension wire that is placed under the skin of the head, neck and shoulder, and a device similar to a cardiac pacemaker is implanted in the chest or stomach.

The device delivers electrical impulses to the leads that go into the brain. These impulses interfere with and block the abnormal nerve signals that cause the symptoms of Parkinson's disease.[10]

Before the procedure, the patient has an MRI (magnetic resonance imaging) or CT scan (computed tomography) to locate the area in the brain where electrical nerve signals generate the Parkinson's symptoms.[11]

The surgery is usually conducted under local rather than general anaesthesia because it's important for the patient to provide feedback when the doctor is finding the right spot to place the electrode. 'If we turn the electric charge on and their tremor stops then we know we're in a pretty good area,' says Dr Bittar. 'We also like to see whether they're getting any side effects. There is no point in fixing someone's tremor when they're getting a severe side effect.'

Some surgeons don't believe that is the case and will perform the procedure while the patient is asleep. But Dr Bittar says, 'The downside of keeping the patient awake is well and truly justified by the potential benefit—the degree of confidence in placing the electrode and giving the patients the best possible chance of a good outcome.'

Patient Peter McWilliam had some fears about remaining awake on the operating table for several hours while doctors probed his brain. 'They gave me a sedative drug that made me forget everything that happened on the table. It was less traumatic than going to the dentist,' he says.

According to Dr Bittar, there is a bit of pain involved. 'We generally try to use more local anaesthetic and sedation to try and keep the patient as comfortable as possible. It's not a procedure without discomfort but that's the price patients pay to increase their chances of getting a good result,' he says.

Dr Bittar has used DBS for more than 150 patients. He says the surgery has become more popular, since its mainstream

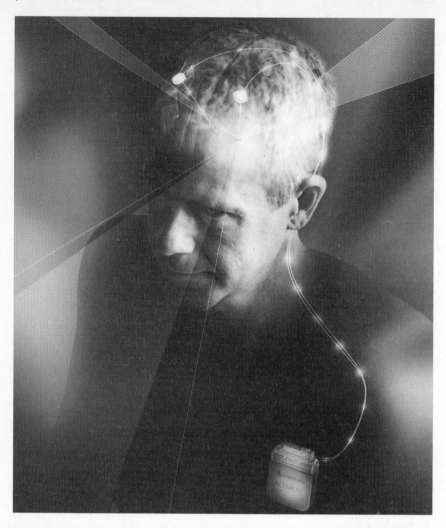

In deep brain stimulation, electrodes are implanted into the brain and attached to a device similar to a cardiac pacemaker, which is implanted into the chest or stomach. Courtesy Medtronic

acceptance several years ago. 'That's partly due to the patients being more aware of its existence and the neurologists being more aware of the potential benefits.'

He says people are seeing better results now than five or ten years ago, as brain scan technology and techniques improve:

One in four or five of my patients will come off medication. On average, they reduce their medications by 30 to 70 per cent.

—Dr Richard Bittar

This surgery and the delivery devices [use of pumps and patches] are not part of the Pharmaceutical Benefits Scheme. As a result many Australians cannot afford to benefit from them.

—HTA, *Help for Today: Hope for Tomorrow*

Deep brain stimulation is a costly operation and not everyone can pay for the treatment.

Even with private health insurance, Peter McWilliam was left about $12,000 out of pocket but he says the results are worth it.

What are the benefits?

The beauty of having the surgery is that many patients who experience bad tremor will get a significant benefit. The amount of time patients spend in an 'off' state, when they are largely frozen, also improves. Generally, doctors say patients will get the same benefit as when they're at their peak on medications, except the dosages have been greatly reduced.

Unfortunately, this also means that if the patient is not benefiting significantly from medication, then they may not benefit from surgery (with the possible exception of tremor management). Surgery is also not appropriate for people with significant thinking and behavioural problems. An age limitation also exists. A review by a neurologist experienced with DBS may be necessary to decide whether surgery would be appropriate.

Another benefit is that DBS does not damage healthy brain tissue and the procedure can be reversed if a cure or more promising treatments are found in the future.

The stimulation from the electrodes can also be reprogrammed if the patient's condition changes, without the need for more surgery. The patient can adjust the voltage—within a safe range that is chosen by the neurologist. However, any major adjustments are left to the neurologist.

Peter McWilliam says the treatment has changed his life. He describes his life of being a virtual recluse before having the surgery. 'Before I couldn't go to a restaurant because I'd put food all over the place. You're effectively eliminated from life. Now my physical movements have calmed right down. I can socialise again.'

The surgery has also enabled him to have a good night's sleep without shaking as hard, and he has had his driver's license returned, giving him much more independence.

What are the risks?
As with all major operations, the patient faces the risk of infection and complications. The risk of infection with DBS is about 3 per cent. There is also a risk of major bleeding, which occurs in 2–3 per cent of cases.

Doctors also say there is a one in 100 chance that a patient will die as a result of the surgery. This would generally occur as a result of a massive haemorrhage or stroke. 'The risks of brain surgery are mildly to moderately increased when compared to most other types of surgery,' says Dr Richard Bittar.

Those risks are higher in the elderly, or in patients who have other underlying medical conditions.

Complications from surgery may include cognitive and visual impairment, swallowing difficulty, seizures and headache.[12] Cognitive problems can occur if there is stimulation of the subthalamic nucleus (STN), a part of the brain which is a popular target for DBS in Parkinson's patients. The risk of this happening is much greater in patients with cognitive problems before surgery, which is why they are assessed by a neuropsychologist beforehand to see whether the target needs to be changed. Dr Bittar says that 'swallowing problems, seizures and visual impairment affects less than 1 per cent of patients as a result of the surgery. Headaches can occur for a few weeks after having the procedure, usually because of air inside the skull. Headaches generally settle completely.'

Who can benefit from DBS?
The benefits of DBS surgery mirror the benefits for medication, but in a more sustained fashion. Not all movement problems in Parkinson's disease will respond to medication, and hence not all movement problems will respond to DBS surgery.

Dr Bittar says surgery doesn't improve things like balance, handwriting or speech. In fact, a patient's voice can become softer with stimulation. Sometimes DBS can aggravate a patient's depression, and for that reason, they are advised to see a psychologist or psychiatrist before surgery so their condition can be carefully managed after surgery. For patients who are cognitively impaired, doctors will try to target another area of their brain, so their thinking processes aren't further affected. Usually the globus pallidus internus (GPi) is chosen instead.

Patients who don't respond well to levodopa medications are generally not suitable for sub-nucleus stimulation. Surgeons also try to avoid operating on patients in the advanced stages of Parkinson's disease, who are not likely to have a reasonable outcome.

Professor Malcolm Horne says the need and indications for DBS typically arise in the middle stage of the disease:

> *Successful DBS is about timing. If it's too late it occurs towards the advanced stages and it exacerbates the problems of disturbed cognition and neuropsychiatry. On the other hand, it shouldn't be performed too soon because it exposes the patient to unnecessary interventional risk. As with all procedures, it is most successful when people with Parkinson's disease are optimally selected and this often*

means 'grooming' patients to be prepared for surgery when the window of opportunity opens.

There is a trend in Australia and around the world to offer DBS to patients with Parkinson's disease at an earlier stage ... before their physical symptoms take hold ... affecting their work and social network.

—Dr Richard Bittar, neurosurgeon

But 33-year-old patient Nerissa Mapes isn't a convert and doesn't believe DBS will be on her horizon any time soon. 'I think it's absolutely terrifying. If I ever thought about it for a millisecond, I always thought of it as an option down the track, when I got really bad.'

Paula Argy says the procedure seems quite frightening, but she wouldn't rule it out. 'I've met some people who've had it done. For some it's been very successful, for others it's not.'

In my view, it's the good, the bad and the ugly. It is good in some sense. But there are bad bits. And my god, there are ugly bits.

—Professor Robert Iansek

Professor Robert Iansek, who runs the Victorian Comprehensive Parkinson Program in Melbourne, is cautious about the benefits of DBS. He believes the procedure is just another alternative to medications for people with advanced Parkinson's disease. And he says it carries risks aside from the ones that come with the actual procedure. There have been examples of personality changes in patients who have had DBS.

Professor Iansek says people who've had the procedure can develop an impulse control disorder as a result of the stimulation. They can become rude, aggressive and extravagant with their money. They often don't see their behaviour as unusual or out of character. Family members bear the brunt of this abnormal behaviour, making them anxious and upset. They often blame these 'personality changes' on DBS. Because stimulation can aggravate a patient's personality, Professor Iansek says the results of DBS may cause relationships to break down.

> *The part of the brain that is stimulated not only regulates mobility but also behaviour, mood and cognition. We have to be very careful that people are cognitively intact before they have the surgery otherwise the stimulation can aggravate pre-existing cognitive deficits. In addition, pre-existing severe depression can sometimes lead to post-operative suicide attempts even if DBS is successful from a movement viewpoint.*

One way of addressing this dilemma is to ensure the patient is fully informed about the risks so they can weigh them up against the benefits of surgery. He says patients in his program are thoroughly educated about the pros and cons of DBS, and it can take some time before they decide to go ahead with surgery.

> *It can take about 12 months, from when we advise people that it might be an option to the time they actually have the surgery. We want them to think very hard about it and understand it, to make sure that's exactly what they want. And we have to be extremely careful to involve the family. They have to be made aware of all the issues. They have to be prepared, so if there are any problems it doesn't come as a surprise and they're not left devastated by the whole process.*

Dr David Heydrick's story

I was 39 and driving home from my neurology practice, and noticed my dominant right finger was slower than my left. A few months later tremor started, followed by micrographia [small handwriting].

After a scan, I came to grips with my diagnosis of Parkinson's. Unfortunately, things went from bad to worse rapidly. I couldn't work, write, drive, button shirts, give talks or even be much of a father to my two boys, including throwing a baseball accurately.

I had reached rock bottom. So in 2005, I went where I originally said I never would: DBS (of the bilateral subthalamic nucleus [STN], staged nine months apart). In hindsight I wish I had done it earlier. I had gone through two miserable years of increasing disability, trying all medications. With DBS, in a matter of months, this was reversed. DBS exceeded my expectations and restored my function and quality of life. I remain off medication. Last month in one week I rode 500 miles [800 kilometres] across Iowa on a regular road bike with my son and the Pedalling for Parkinson's Team. This would not have been imaginable two years ago.

For about a third of bilateral DBS recipients, the most troubling post-DBS symptom is speech dysfunction. I trade off my voice for tremor control. I can knock out my tremor if I turn up the voltage but I can't talk. During my bike ride in Iowa I turned DBS off for four hours of intense riding on a tandem bike: the exercise quieted the tremor and my voice was normal. It was a great day. Not all DBS patients have speech dysfunction so possibly it is electrode placement–dependent. I have heard of surgeons testing for voice dysfunction during the surgery, which I would advocate.

My balance was obviously affected. I would reach over to a counter and fall over. This was entirely new and directly related to having bilateral DBS. Better understanding of anatomy relating to balance problems would be quite beneficial for electrode placement and/or programming. Walking different directions on a treadmill and doing tai chi (though not at the same time!) helped with this.

—Adapted from Dr David Heydrick's speech
on 21 August 2006 at Bethesda, Maryland, USA

The latest DBS research

US research suggests DBS provides better symptom control than medical therapy for patients of all ages. A recent study surveyed 255 patients, a quarter of whom were aged more than 70 years. Of these, 121 patients had deep brain stimulation, while 134 received the best medical therapy. The results were measured after six months.

Patients who had DBS experienced an extra 4.6 hours a day of good motor control six months after surgery. The DBS group also reported greater improvements in quality of life than those on medical therapy.

The bad news? DBS patients reported 659 moderate or severe adverse events, such as infection from surgery, falls, gait disturbance and dyskinesias. In contrast, the medical therapy patients reported 236 adverse events. More falls were recorded in the DBS group, and behavioural problems, such as depression, confusion and anxiety were higher.[13]

Ablative neurosurgery

Another surgical treatment is ablative surgery, in which a select region of the brain is destroyed to control some of the symptoms. The area of the brain is heated, using radio frequency radiation or high frequency electric currents (thermocoagulation). The problem with this procedure is that once the tissue is destroyed it cannot be replaced and the side effects cannot be adjusted.[14]

Experts suggest this procedure is now rarely done in Australia, because it has largely been replaced by DBS which is a more recent development. The use of ablative surgery is generally restricted to those people who are not suitable for deep brain stimulation and other highly selected cases.[15]

Radiosurgery

Radiosurgery is a means of focusing high-energy radiation onto a very localised part of the brain with the aim of destroying the tissue. It's very successful in treating brain tumours and blood vessel malformations in the brain.

A study of 183 Parkinson's patients who underwent radiosurgery found that about 83 per cent were almost or completely cured of their tremors seven years later. The results were presented at a conference in November 2009.[16]

In reporting the study, Dr Rufus Mark of the Joe Arrington Cancer Center and Texas Tech University, said:

> The study shows that radiosurgery is an effective and safe method of getting rid of tremors caused by Parkinson's disease with outcomes that favourably compare to both deep-brain stimulation and radiofrequency in tremor relief and risk of complications at seven years after treatment.
>
> In view of these long-term results, this non-invasive procedure should be considered as a primary treatment option for tremors that are hard to treat.

Complementary treatments

Complementary and alternative medicines are a big market in Australia. About half of the general population turn to non-conventional medicine to treat problems and improve their wellbeing.[17] But the truth is there is no scientific evidence to demonstrate the effectiveness of many of these products and therapies that carry promises of 'relief' or even a 'cure'.

However, studies have shown support for the benefits of some complementary therapies for particular ailments. For example, there is evidence that the use of acupuncture can help with dental pain and the nausea and vomiting associated with chemotherapy. St John's wort is a popular herbal remedy for mild depression, and gingko biloba might help in the treatment of dementia.[18]

It is important to note that the industry is not as regulated as conventional medicine, so patients need to do some research before using non-conventional medicine. Parkinson's patients should always speak to a neurologist or their doctor about the benefits or risks of treatment.

Paula Argy takes three magnesium (chelate) tablets to reduce cramping and muscular problems. She takes the tablets at night so they don't interact with her Parkinson's medication during the day. Paula also takes large amounts of fish oil, as well as tablets of evening primrose oil and zinc for her general wellbeing. Her doctors say she is wasting her money. But she says studies do point to their benefits. 'For me, complementary therapy is a nutritional thing, which makes me feel better.'

A Melbourne patient reveals his remarkable journey in a book called *Stop Parkin' and Start Livin'*. John Coleman claims complementary therapies have helped him recover from Parkinson's disease, and remain symptom free. John says he was very unhappy with Western medical practitioners who were treating his Parkinson's disease and decided to pursue other options. He considered homeopathy, aquahydration formulas, Bowen therapy, craniosacral therapy, flower essences, counselling, meditation and spiritual development. He maintains there is 'no cure for Parkinson's disease. But given my own experience and that of a very few individuals around the world, there is a way to recover.'[19]

When seeking help from any complementary therapist, patients should find out:[20]

- their qualifications
- whether they are registered with a professional body
- their experience in treating people with Parkinson's disease
- if there is any evidence of treatment benefits for Parkinson's patients
- if this evidence is independently validated

- the potential risks for individual health conditions, including the interaction of complementary medicines with conventional Parkinson's disease medicines
- how long it will be before benefits are seen
- what the cost of treatment will be and if the treatment is eligible for refunds under private health insurance.

Acupuncture

Acupuncture is a form of traditional Chinese medicine in which thin needles or acupoints are placed on carefully chosen points of the body. Anecdotal evidence suggests acupuncture can improve some Parkinson's symptoms, including tremor, walking difficulties, rigidity and pain. Many people also find that acupuncture increases their energy levels, induces relaxation, improves appetite and sleep, and provides an overall sense of wellbeing.[21]

Alexander technique

Patients learn techniques to improve their posture and muscle activity. A randomised clinical trial showed that Alexander technique can improve self-assessed disability of people with Parkinson's compared with no intervention or massage. The benefit lasted six months.[22]

Homeopathy

Homeopaths prescribe highly diluted natural substances with the aim of treating the individual, not just the illness. Homeopathy does not cause side effects or addiction, but you must always alert your doctor to any homeopathic medicines you take as these could interact with Parkinson's medications.[23]

Massage

This may be a good way of relieving stiffness and muscular pain. A small pilot study has suggested that massage therapy is superior to progressive muscle relaxation exercise to improve the activities of daily life for people with Parkinson's.[24]

Reflexology

Reflexology is based on massaging certain areas of the foot to influence the body's inner organs. There is no evidence that it has a specific effect on Parkinson's, but reflexology can promote relaxation and improve circulation. It may also be helpful to off-set some of the side effects of traditional Parkinson's treatments. For example, it can stimulate the saliva glands and tear ducts, the actions of which are often suppressed by Parkinson's medications. Reflexology may also help to relieve constipation.[25]

Dietary supplements

While the market for vitamins is booming, there is no compelling evidence that vitamins or other dietary supplements help treat Parkinson's disease.

The only exception is an anti-oxidant called co-enzyme Q10. A trial conducted in several centres showed that co-enzyme Q10 is safe and well tolerated at dosages of up to 1200mg per day. The trial showed that less disability developed in patients who were assigned the supplement compared with those receiving a placebo. The benefit was greatest for patients who received the highest dosage. Co-enzyme Q10 appears to slow the progressive deterioration of function in Parkinson's disease, but these results need to be confirmed in a larger study.[26]

> *I don't swear by supplements. I don't know if they make a difference in the sense of relieving my Parkinson's. But I feel better. That's why I do it.*
>
> —Paula Argy

Sydney homeopath Deborah Rayfield says complementary therapy can work alongside conventional medicine. 'We would say give it a try. It can be extraordinarily effective and many people do benefit,' she says.

> *If I saw five people with Parkinson's disease, those five*
> *will probably walk out the door with different homeopathic*
> *remedies. They're tailored to the individual.*
> *We have medicines that come from all three kingdoms.*
> *Animal, plant and mineral kingdoms. In Parkinson's, it's*
> *often remedies in the mineral kingdom that can help.*
> *People talk about the placebo effect with homeopathy. And*
> *I have no problem with that. If people feel better just by*
> *talking, why not?*
>
> *Even meditation is important. To rest and relax is really*
> *essential. We don't do that well enough in our society. Plenty*
> *of air and light around you, that's important. Especially [if*
> *you work in] offices with airconditioning.*

Clinical psychologist Chris Basten is sceptical of the perceived benefits of complementary therapies, but says they shouldn't do any harm, so long as patients seek medical advice before trying them.

> *If somebody thinks they're doing their nervous system*
> *the greatest good by doing a combination of tai chi and*
> *breathing exercises and taking a certain extract, good on*
> *them. So long as they're taking their levodopa as well.*

Professor Rob Iansek says patients have every right to choose other options, but they need to ensure it doesn't cause financial hardship. He comments that:

> *If it doesn't cost the person too much money and it doesn't*
> *cause many side effects and if they feel it helps them, then*
> *by all means let them try it. In Canada, they investigated the*

'placebo' effect and it actually showed that if patients thought they were going to get better, they made more dopamine. There is a very strong placebo effect in all the drug trials in people with Parkinson's disease. Some people want to try complementary therapies without conventional drugs, but eventually they realise it's very hard to function unless they use mainstay treatments.

You pay a neurologist for the best advice you can get. I wouldn't recommend anything but straight medical treatment.
             —John Silk, diagnosed with Parkinson's in his 60s

More information on complementary therapies

Better Health
    www.betterhealth.vic.gov.au
    This website explains the types of complementary therapies available.

European Parkinson's Disease Association
    www.epda.eu.com
    Click on 'Rewrite tomorrow' for information on Parkinson's including complementary therapies

Natural Therapy Pages
    www.naturaltherapypages.com.au
    This site is the central online catalogue for complementary therapy in Australia. It has information on therapists, associations and schools.

Parkinson's Disease Society
    www.parkinsons.org.au
    Download their booklet *Complementary therapies and Parkinson's disease* for more information.

4. STAGES OF PARKINSON'S

How Parkinson's develops

People who are diagnosed with Parkinson's disease often think the disease takes hold quickly and that rapid decline is inevitable.

Unlike many other illnesses, such as advanced cancer or motor neurone disease, where the prognosis may be grim because treatment options are limited, this isn't the case with Parkinson's disease. Many patients manage their condition for well over two decades, but decline is inevitable unless new treatments are found. Actor Michael J. Fox, who was diagnosed in 1991, is one of many patients who has lived with the disease for many years.

> When I was diagnosed, I was determined to absorb the blow, suck up all the fear, pain, confusion and doubt and be grateful that a small group of friends and family were there to catch whatever spilled over.[1]

Peter McWilliam, 67, from Sydney, was diagnosed in 1992, a year after Michael J. Fox. He has managed his symptoms by taking medication, but over time his doses have increased because the drugs became ineffective and unreliable. So Peter took the plunge and had surgery. That option proved to be his lifeline, as it has given him renewed independence.

Neurologists say some people become fearful about taking drugs when they are first diagnosed, especially younger patients. Anxiety sets in and they want to see whether they can 'beat it' or 'stay the same' without having treatment. Dr Victor Fung says they're afraid that medications will mask the true extent of their disease. However, avoiding medication does not usually help because the disease does progress and symptoms become worse over time. Studies have shown that delaying the onset of medication for too long results in a worse outcome: from falls and other consequences of poorly treated disease. Some people fear medication is harmful but there is no evidence to support that. Dr Fung says it's better to take medications to reverse the symptoms and improve quality of life.

But the experts also say that everyone is different and there is no way of measuring exactly how someone's disease will progress. One thing's for sure, the disease manifests slowly and there is time for someone to adapt and make changes to their life, rather than being caught unaware.

> *Expect major change in five- to ten-year intervals.*
> —Dr Victor Fung, neurologist

Most people who develop symptoms in their late 30s or early 40s might have a lot of problems with motor control, but won't develop dementia until much later: they're likely to reach their 60s or 70s without developing dementia. About 30 per cent of patients develop dementia, and the older they are, the higher the risk.[2]

Early stage

In the early stages of the disease, treatment is not generally required if the patient's symptoms aren't affecting their daily life.[3] But once symptoms start to interfere with activities, specialists recommend starting either levodopa or a dopamine agonist (see Chapter 3). The latter is often preferred because dopamine agonists have been shown to delay the onset of motor fluctuations and reduce the incidence of involuntary movements (or dyskinesias). The increased risk of side effects from dopamine agonists compared with L-dopa, may mean that elderly patients are better off commencing therapy with L-dopa than agonists.

The advantage of starting on levodopa is that it provides greater symptom relief more quickly. Many patients fear that levodopa may be toxic, which has been ruled out, or that early treatment may dampen the impact of treatment later in the disease. But there is no definitive evidence that this class of drug affects the way the disease runs its course.

However, experts say there is a 'honeymoon' period when movement problems can be reversed and function return to normal for many patients. This period depends on the stage of disease at diagnosis, and the honeymoon period can be missed if the therapy is delayed until after a person's disability takes hold.

Most patients in the early stages of the disease will experience continuous relief from movement problems, despite only taking two or three doses of medication each day. This amount of medication is quite normal for someone who is newly diagnosed.

Early stage

- Movement problems may require medication.
- A dopamine agonist drug is often preferred to delay the onset of motor fluctuations (particularly in younger patients).
- There is generally a 'honeymoon period' when movement problems can be reversed with medication.
- Most patients will experience relief by taking two to three doses of medication each day.

Middle stage

After three to five years, most patients start to notice changes in their ability to control movement throughout the day. Fluctuations in motor function will affect about half of patients within five years, and almost all patients will experience a roller-coaster effect within ten years. The roller-coaster effect refers to times during the day and week when it is harder to retain control over movement because of the unstable effect of medication as the disease progresses.

Problems in controlling movement can occur when patients don't have enough dopamine stimulation from their medication, which is considered the 'off' period. When patients achieve a good motor response with medication it's called the 'on' period, or they could be somewhere in-between.

The first sign that someone is about to experience the 'roller-coaster' effect is usually when 'off' symptoms emerge towards the end of a dose. This is also known as the 'wearing off' effect. Initially, this might occur during the night or on waking. This is because the patient has gone without medication for a long period through the night. Neurologist Dr Scott Whyte says in the early stages of the disease the brain is still capable of making enough dopamine overnight, so a patient may be able to move freely without medication in the morning. This sleep benefit usually only lasts for a relatively short period during the day and medication will then be needed to allow good movement to continue. In time, this sleep benefit is reduced and finally lost, resulting in a need for medication to be given before getting out of bed, or throughout the evening to allow movement once the person has woken up. At first, a slow-release L-dopa based medication before going to bed may be sufficient for someone to move properly during the night and morning. As time goes by, longer acting drugs such as a dopamine agonist may be needed.

Later, the 'off' periods may become unpredictable. Dr

Whyte says this is probably due to a number of reasons, including changes in the function of the bowel and alterations of the sensitivity of nerve cells to medication. The changes in bowel function result in a slower and less predictable passage of medication from the stomach to the small bowel. Medication is not absorbed in the stomach and must pass to the small bowel to be absorbed. This is a problem particularly if medication is taken with food or soon after a meal, as fluid passes more slowly to the small bowel when the stomach is full. This may result in apparent medication failure when taken with food or soon after meals. Taking medication half an hour before meals, or one and a half hours after a meal, may help if this is a problem. Stress and anxiety can also trigger a wearing-off effect. Many patients eventually develop involuntary movements despite being 'on', if the amount of dopamine stimulation peaks above a certain level.

Medication failure at the end of a dose is most often managed by taking levodopa more frequently, or adding other medications to extend the life of levodopa.

As well as experiencing a return of symptoms, many patients eventually develop dyskinesias in response to dopamine medications. They can range from mild to severe and can lead to falls. The movements are managed initially by reducing individual doses of levodopa and increasing the frequency of doses, or adding a dopamine agonist. If this doesn't work, then adding amantadine will reduce or sometimes remove peak-dose dyskinesias in about 60 per cent of patients.

Middle stage

- Half of patients will experience motor fluctuations within five years.
- Many people will develop involuntary movements—a side effect of their dopamine medication.
- Motor fluctuations are best managed by changing their medication regime.

- Problems with freezing (akinesia) can occur at night or in the morning.
- Cognition, behaviour and mood changes may also occur in the middle stage of the disease.

Late stage

In the later stages of the disease, 10 to 15 years after diagnosis, it's common for motor, psychiatric and cognitive problems to develop despite the use of medication. 'In this later stage, the disease spreads out from the mainly movement-related areas that use dopamine as their main chemical signal, to other areas of the brain that use a wider variety of chemicals than dopamine,' says Dr Whyte. Medications aimed at changing dopamine levels, or drugs that may look like dopamine, are understandably not effective. Some of the features that typically do not respond to the standard medications include balancing, swallowing, thinking, bladder, bowel and blood pressure problems. As these problems become more common in later disease, it is understandable when the typical Parkinson's medications appear less effective. When this happens, other drugs and strategies may help. For example, strategies to assist with swallowing may reduce the chance of a person developing pneumonia.

Typical Parkinson's medications may continue to produce a benefit to movement, but are more often limited by physical responses such as poor balance. For example, a patient may be able to stand and walk when the medication turns them 'on', but they may need a stick or frame to stop them from falling due to poor balance.

In an Australian study, 130 people with Parkinson's disease were followed up over 15 years. The study found that a majority remained in the early stages of the disease for a considerable amount of time, before moving to the next stages or even dying from other causes before Parkinson's disease became more severe. Dr Victor Fung says a minority of patients die from Parkinson's-related complications, and the average life expectancy of someone with Parkinson's disease is generally the same as that of people who do not have the disease.[4]

Late stage

- Walking is limited and the patient can become incapacitated and unable to live alone.
- While the average life expectancy of a Parkinson's disease patient is generally the same as for people without the disease, in the late stages the disease can cause complications, such as choking, pneumonia and falls, that can lead to death.[5]
- It may take 20 years or more for the symptoms of Parkinson's disease to progress fully. In some people, however, the disease may progress more slowly or rapidly. There is no way to predict what course the disease will take for an individual.

John Ball's story

As far as my goals are concerned: I know now as a 64-year-old that I will not be piloting rocket ships to the stars, but I need not blame that on Parkinson's. After all, I don't see anyone else going there either. And I know that I'll never conquer Mount Everest, but I'd be lying if I blamed that on Parkinson's as well. And finally, I never made the Olympic team, but I haven't given up entirely on calling myself an athlete. I haven't really given up on any of my dreams: I've just had to reshape them. Oh, I still find a way to fly occasionally, even if it's just remote-control airplanes. And I have learned that by carefully gathering my resources I can still scale smaller mountains, and by planning strategically and training hard I can still run. The best thing I've learned is that by setting these challenging but achievable goals I can help and inspire others to achieve their goals.

As to my dreams of scaling the highest peaks, in the fall of 2004, I climbed Cirque Peak with my older brother Jim and his girlfriend Nancy. It's a 13,000 footer [4000 metres] in the Sierra Nevadas of California. It was Nancy's first summit and preparation for climbing Mt Kilimanjaro. As we finished the descent, she said: 'That was the hardest thing I've ever done.' I knew she would have to revise that after Kilimanjaro, but I was very glad to have helped her get ready for a truly extraordinary effort.

And my Olympic dream? Well, this spring I ran my 13th consecutive Los Angeles Marathon and finished [with a time of] 4:49:22. Certainly not an Olympic-level performance but I was in the top third of my age group. Since then I've run both the Catalina Island Marathon and the San Francisco Marathon, bringing my total to 19 complete marathons. The course on Catalina goes up and down over 4,000-feet [1200-metre] elevation change, so it took over five hours, but I finished San Francisco in four hours, 23 minutes and 22 seconds. I also clocked a sub-two-hour half-marathon earlier this year. I hadn't gone that fast in quite a few years. My wife says I'm not getting any younger, but at least I'm picking up a little speed. You may wonder how this is possible since I've been living with Parkinson's for over 35 years? Well, believe me, there are times when I wonder as well.

I've lived with Parkinson's for over half my life, so what have I learned from it?

Lesson #1: I am not defined by my disease. I have Parkinson's, but it doesn't have me. It's just something that happened to me, like having blue eyes or losing my hair. It is just an obstacle to overcome and I choose whether to be a victim or victor. Here's what I decided to do:

Take care of myself. I know that sounds selfish, but it's like they say on the airlines about the oxygen mask. You won't be able to take care of others if you don't take care of yourself first. That means living a healthy lifestyle. A healthy lifestyle includes eating a good diet, not overeating, not drinking to excess, getting as much sleep as possible, keeping stress to a minimum and all the other good habits that healthy people live by. It also means learning which foods impact on my medications, and when to take my meals so they do not interfere. And most importantly, it means paying attention to my level of fitness and staying strong.

Take part in the community. This took me some time to figure out because I was quite successful in dealing with my Parkinson's by myself. It took me several years to figure out that I really wasn't dealing with it by myself. Everyone around me at home and at work was dealing with it as well. None of us with chronic illness can deal with it in isolation because it affects everyone around us, particularly those close to us.

The third thing I did was to identify Parkinson's as a cause worth living for and dedicating myself to it. It wasn't enough for me just to join the community—I needed to become an advocate for it. I believe you really can't make a difference if you don't show up … so I try to be a part of everything that has a bearing on the PD community.

Lesson #2: I also learned to decide for myself what's really important for me to keep in my life and what to give up. I loved riding motorcycles and flying airplanes, for example. And when I was diagnosed, the doctor said I had to give up my aircraft medical certificate and he told me to get rid of my motorcycle. I did so because I didn't know any better. I went ten years without riding or flying, and then learned that I didn't really need to. Ten years after my diagnosis, I was still able to pass a flight medical exam and my flying privileges were restored. I learned to decide for myself what I can or can't do. That doesn't mean I just ignore the advice of my doctors or my family when they say I shouldn't do something, because some things are genuinely risky because of PD, like woodworking. Yes, I lost part of my thumb, but I'm going to keep my wood shop going as long as possible.

Lesson #3: I learned how to adjust my targets and expectations as my capabilities change. I know that Parkinson's has eaten away at my productivity. I know I'm no longer able to multi-task like I used to. I recognise that I am less able to get everything done in a day than I was 10 or 15 years ago. Hey, I can blame it on PD or I can blame it on being 64, but it doesn't make any difference; nor does it do any good to shift away the responsibility. It may also mean that I have to be honest with myself and ask for help when I need it.

Lesson #4: I need to keep growing and taking on new skills and challenges. Our world is changing all around us constantly and I want to be able to grow with those changes. That means I have to have the right tools in my tool kit. What I mean is that we have all assembled over the course of our lives the habits of thought and action that make us comfortable in handling life on a daily basis. I think it's important to know as much as I can about this Parkie that lives within me. That's why I say, 'It's not the guy with the most toys that wins; It's the guy with the most tools.' If I keep all these tools at my fingertips and keep them sharp and ready to use, how can I not succeed?

Lesson #5: Parkie can be a devious companion to deal with and he doesn't always come straight at you. I'm talking about depression. It's part of PD, and for many of us, it is part of life. I'm not just talking about having the blues; I'm talking about being clinically and chronically sick. Depression can strip you of your most comfortable tools. It can take away your logic and fog your perception of reality. It can dull your senses and blur your feelings to such an extent that you mistake pain for pleasure and abuse for love. I found I needed to expand my doctor's circle to include a psychologist and needed to include an antidepressant in my medications list for a while. I also enlisted the help of friends and family to correct my misimpressions and help me see reality. I also needed to cast aside those feelings of guilt and unworthiness. It wasn't my fault for having PD, and I wasn't to blame for being depressed. It's just another symptom of this disease. It isn't our fault for being sick, but we do have to take responsibility for our recovery.

Lesson #6: Looking at it realistically, I would have to admit that the challenge of PD is a mixed blessing. Yes, it's a sly and challenging companion to live with, and a constant threat to wreak havoc on my future, but I have learned so many things I might have missed had it not slowed me down and made me aware of what was at stake. I might have missed the many incredible friendships and the truly wonderful people I have met because of it. A year ago, I gave a lecture on PD at Whittier College and afterward a student asked if I thought my life was better or worse because of Parkinson's. I had to admit that I am very happy with my life.

—Extract from John Ball's speech at the Parkinson's Congress in Sydney, 2008. John was formally diagnosed in 1983, aged 39. His book *Living Well, Running Hard* details his experiences with the disease.

5. Coping with Daily Life

A person with Parkinson's is more likely to fall because they freeze or try to turn while walking as opposed to tripping over a cord on the floor. Sometimes, when a person with PD starts falling over a lot, families and others assume environmental factors are to blame.
—Professor Meg Morris, physiotherapist

One of the biggest hurdles for people with Parkinson's is dealing with mobility problems, especially in the later stages of the disease. Experts believe patients should be taught strategies earlier on before symptoms become worse. There are practical tools so people can avoid freezing on the spot, and to reduce their risk of falling. This chapter will look at the benefits of various strategies such as exercise, and will address issues that affect daily living such as communication and nutrition. Lastly, there are tips on what people can do around the home to make their life more manageable. This can only work with the help of experts, who can address these issues more extensively and tailor programs to suit individual needs.

Mobility, falls and freezing

People who have Parkinson's disease are more prone to falls because of the poor balance, muscle weakness and freezing episodes that result from the disease. Despite the use of medication to address these symptoms, up to 68 per cent of people who have Parkinson's disease will fall, and up to 46 per cent will suffer repeated falls each year.[1]

While it's often thought that people who are in an advanced stage of the disease are more likely to fall and injure themselves, this group is generally not as active as middle-stage patients, who tend to be more vulnerable to tripping because they're still very mobile.

Professor Malcolm Horne says that falls are often a sign that someone is entering the advanced stages of disease, when treatments are no longer working and other parts of the brain are also beginning to fail. He says, 'People won't use walking aids because they see [that] as giving into the disease rather than seeing it as a way of keeping independent and fighting it.'

Falls can cause devastating injury and pain, which is why they are one of the major reasons for Parkinson's patients being admitted to hospital.[2]

> *People with Parkinson's disease have a higher incidence of falling and fracturing their hip than the elderly population. When they do fall, they don't tend to use their arms to balance themselves in the same way as elderly people who don't have the disease.*
>
> —Dr Colleen Canning, physiotherapist

Who is at risk of falling?
People who are prone to falling:

- have suffered a previous fall
- have more severe disease
- have leg muscle weakness
- have reduced balance
- experience freezing of gait.

Dr Colleen Canning says people are likely to fall when their footsteps get shorter, and their head and shoulders get ahead of their feet. Appropriate Parkinson's medication and the use of cueing strategies can help reduce freezing. Walking aides such as sticks and frames may also help.

Home-based exercise to reduce falls

Researchers in the United Kingdom carried out the first large trial to measure the effectiveness of a home-based exercise program for people who have Parkinson's disease and repeatedly fall.

A physiotherapist visited patients weekly at home. The exercises included muscle strengthening, balance training and walking. The physiotherapist also taught patients strategies for preventing falls and measures to initiate walking. After the initial six-week treatment period, the patients were encouraged to continue with their exercises, and any problems were discussed with a physiotherapist.

Findings from the trial showed that people with Parkinson's disease tended to experience lower rates of falling when they undertook a program of home-based exercises delivered by a physiotherapist and learned strategies for safe movement. Fewer people who took part in the program had near falls or repeated near falls than the group in the study who did not take part in the exercise program. The patients who had less severe Parkinson's disease also benefited more from the exercise program than those whose disease was more advanced. The researchers recommended further trials of this type of intervention earlier in the disease progression, before the patient began to experience severe balance problems.[3]

There is some evidence to suggest exercise and other interventions mentioned below can help reduce falls. Other studies have also shown specific programs can improve the three risk factors for falls: muscle weakness, less secure balance and freezing.

Freezing occurs when a patient's feet feel glued to the floor, and it takes a lot of effort for them to start moving. Their surroundings can worsen their predicament. Moving through doorways, making turns and cluttered rooms all prove to be major obstacles for Parkinson's patients. Neurologist Dr Scott Whyte says one theory on the cause is that people freeze when their concentration is taken away from the task of moving. He says a nearby obstacle such as a doorway or table can be too distracting. Strategies that put the focus back on movement, for example counting or marching when approaching a door, or moving an obstacle away from the walkway can prove very effective in reducing the likelihood of freezing. Many other strategies are available to help overcome freezing episodes, and a review by a Parkinson's management team may be very helpful.

> *If it's a tight doorway I can't get through. It's bizarre but I just freeze. My brain stops. The barrier on either side just stops me. When I go through a crowd I'll need someone to guide me through, otherwise I sometimes freeze.*
> —Paula Argy, young mother with Parkinson's disease

Managing freezing

External cues, such as putting strips of marking tape on the floor, stepping over a stick, walking to a rhythm or getting reminders from their partner to take off with a big step, can help greatly.[4] The value of these measures is currently being investigated by researchers in Australia.

> *Automatic control is lost or diminished in people with Parkinson's disease. Instead of getting big steps at a nice regular rhythm, what you tend to get is shorter steps at a faster frequency but with an overall slow speed. Cueing strategies help get a person's attention back onto walking.*
> —Dr Colleen Canning

Paula Argy has used some of these techniques to overcome everyday hurdles. She describes them as '100 per cent helpful'. When she's having an 'off' period while shopping, for instance, Paula looks down at her feet and counts the squares on the floor to enable her to start moving. Paula says that, if she looks up, she's more inclined to freeze. In another episode, Paula was filmed by a doctor to document her symptoms while she was off her medication. 'There were tiles on the floor in the hallway and the minute I looked at the tiles I could walk. It's amazing how the brain works like that,' she said.

Paula has even used audio cues to help her move. She'll use the beat to a piece of music to get started. 'It just works. It gets me through.'

Carrying a miniature metronome on a belt can also help. The device, used by some musicians in their practice sessions to maintain an even tempo, also helps people with Parkinson's to initiate steps and maintain a walking pattern.

Another technique Paula has found useful is running. If she gets stuck, she finds it easier to run than walk to destinations—whether it's to her bedroom or to a book club in her suburb.

Physiotherapist Professor Meg Morris says there is a biological reason why running works for some people. 'The thought of running comes from the front part of the brain, or frontal cortex.' Deciding to run instead of walk avoids the region of the brain that is affected by Parkinson's, which is the basal ganglia. The basal ganglia, which is about the size of a walnut, rests deep within the brain and controls automatic movement. 'So if someone thinks of an automatic task like walking, which runs through the basal ganglia, their action is compromised.'

Professor Morris says that, in helping Parkinson's disease patients manage their mobility problems, 'We try and avoid automatic movements because they're the ones that shrink and become slow, and we consciously think about movements to use the frontal cortex. Paula's desire to run gets away from the basal ganglia which is not working properly.'

Professor Morris says some of her patients find other ways of avoiding freezing episodes, such as taking a few steps backwards or sideways. She says:

> In Parkinson's, the architecture of the brain is not damaged, unlike stroke or head injuries. It's the petrol that runs the system, the neurotransmitters, that's lacking. What we need to do is trick the brain to use the frontal cortex or other areas not affected by Parkinson's to control movement.
>
> So using vision or auditory cues, like a musical beat or tapping your hand, or stepping over an upturned walking stick, will get the front part of the brain to trigger movement.

But for these strategies to be effective, they should be taught early on while a person is still able to plan, think and practise. Then those skills can be used further down the track when they're needed.

Cueing training to manage mobility

A European trial, the largest of its kind and involving 153 patients, found that nine sessions of cueing training in the home helped patients manage their gait, freezing and balance issues.

Patients were given a prototype cueing device (which is not commercially available). The device gave patients three options: an auditory function (a beep delivered through an earpiece), a visual function (light flashes attached to a pair of glasses) and somatosensory (pulsed vibrations delivered by a miniature cylinder worn under the wristband). The cueing device aimed to improve step length and walking speed, prevent freezing episodes and improve balance.

In addition, a home physiotherapy program also provided other instructions to help patients deal with different environments. The tasks completed during the study included walking over various surfaces and for long distances, dual-tasking while walking, stepping sideways and backwards, and cues to help with turns and manoeuvres in tight places and doorways.

The researchers concluded that cueing training in the patient's home had a small and specific benefit for managing gait and freezing in Parkinson's patients.[5]

Current research

An Australian research team, led by Professor Meg Morris at the University of Melbourne, was awarded more than $800,000 from the US-based Michael J. Fox Foundation in 2006. The aim of the study was to determine whether physical therapy approaches can prevent falls and enhance mobility in people with Parkinson's. About 200 people are participating in the study. They are doing strengthening exercises using a weighted vest and a variety of techniques to retrain the mind to carry out tasks that were previously automatic. The results of the study are not yet known.

A similar study, led by Dr Colleen Canning of the University of Sydney, will involve 230 patients with Parkinson's disease. It will help to determine whether exercise can reduce the number of falls in these patients.

This program targets three risk factors: reduced balance, poor leg muscle strength and freezing. They are required to do weight-bearing balance and strengthening exercises, three times a week for six months. Cueing strategies will also be used to address freezing problems. The exercise program sets out different degrees of challenges, from simply standing with feet together and then turning, to standing on one leg and skipping over obstacles. Strengthening exercises will include the use of weighted vests.

How exercise can help

Animal studies have shown that exercise has protective benefits against the onset of symptoms in Parkinson's disease.

—*Molecular Brain Research Journal*, 2005

Physiotherapists recommend that patients keep up their normal exercise routine after they have been diagnosed with Parkinson's disease. While the benefits of exercise are clear, it's still not certain what type is best for people with Parkinson's disease.

Professor Meg Morris says when a person is newly diagnosed, their symptoms are usually not too severe. They might have some slowness of movement, and the size of their steps might become smaller. For this group of patients, the sorts of exercise that can help are things like golf, tai chi, yoga, aerobics and pilates method exercise. She says boosting the level of physical activity can help with breathing, posture, balance and general fitness. In the early stages of the disease, a good way for patients to maintain fitness is to walk for half an hour, three times a week. Some people also find strength training useful in keeping their muscles strong. For example, using a weighted belt to add resistance. 'The person has to realise that, more than ever, physical activity and exercise are important and it's good to choose activities that are going to be enjoyable and sustainable over time.' Professor Morris says:

Don't give up on your exercise or physical activity because you've been given a diagnosis of Parkinson's. It's important to make it more of a priority, rather than less of a priority.

For someone who is in the middle or advanced stages of the disease, it's vital to seek guidance from a trained health professional on the best form of physical activity. That way, the person can be assessed on how well they move and whether their balance is compromised. Professor Meg Morris says people in the middle to advanced stages can benefit from movement strategy training, progressive resistance strengthening exercises and dancing.

Observational studies have shown that pole striding or Nordic walking improves mobility. Treadmill walking is also beneficial. However, most of these studies have been carried out under intense supervision. Treadmill use may become more difficult and even hazardous in later stages of the disease.

Tai chi appears to be an appropriate, safe and effective form of exercise for some people with mild or moderate forms of the disease. This ancient martial art uses meditation and breathing techniques in a series of slow, relaxing moves. Tai chi was tested on 33 people who had Parkinson's disease in the United States. They took part in twice-weekly tai chi sessions, over 13 weeks. The tai chi group improved over that time more than another group, which received no intervention. People who did tai chi improved with their gait, balance and functional mobility.[6]

Dancing is another alternative form of exercise that is being investigated because pilot studies point to benefits. Dance is performed to music, which may serve as an external cue to help facilitate movement. Dance also teaches specific strategies. For example, people who learn Argentine tango learn how to walk backwards, which people with Parkinson's disease have difficulty doing. Dancing also helps with balance, particularly if dancing with a partner, and by responding to dynamic surrounds. Other studies have also shown that people who have danced throughout their lives have better balance and less variable gait than non-dancers. A comparison of tango, waltz and foxtrot, tai chi and no intervention suggests that participating in any of the dance activities gave superior results compared with no exercise.[7]

Preliminary studies in Perth have shown that pilates is effective in maintaining posture. Pilates is an exercise system that focuses on strengthening the core muscles of the body and improving trunk stability. It combines movements based on gymnastics, yoga, dance and martial arts. It concentrates on activating the deep abdominal muscles to help support the lumbar spine. Liam Johnson, from the Centre for Neuromuscular and Neurological Disorder at the University of Western Australia, conducted a pilot study of the effects of a six-week Pilates training program for people with Parkinson's disease. Those who took part showed significant functional balance and mobility improvements.

Tandem cycling showed surprising results for an American doctor affected by Parkinson's disease. Neurologist David Heydrick experienced a dramatic improvement in his symptoms when he took up tandem cycling with a friend, neuroscientist Jay Alberts. After riding 80 kilometres across Iowa, Heydrick's tremor was greatly reduced and his handwriting, for instance, improved dramatically. In a video the pair shot before the ride, Heydrick's hand shook wildly, but afterward it was steady. Alberts told ABC's *Good Morning America* television program that the results suggest there was some change in the central nervous system or the brain function, and maybe they had found a method of exercise that actually treats the disease rather than treats some of the symptoms. Alberts decided to carry out a small trial at Ohio's Cleveland Clinic to test whether eight weeks of forced exercise on a tandem bike could reduce Parkinson's disease symptoms. He told the ABC 'there was a 35 per cent improvement in motor functioning for those patients who did the forced exercise compared to the voluntary exercise'. The improvement lasted four weeks, and then dwindled. Following that study, brain scans were carried out, comparing a patient on medication and a patient who exercised. The same brain regions were activated in both. Alberts hopes further research will help provide more clues as to why tandem cycling seems to produce benefits.[8]

Experts say it's best to adopt an exercise program that suits the patient, with the help of a physiotherapist, occupational therapist or skilled nurse practitioner. If someone suffers from cognitive impairment, then the program can't be too mentally challenging. For example, if a person struggles to do two things at once they should be advised against talking while they walk or else they risk falling (see the next section for a discussion on this).

It's important that an exercise program is reviewed regularly so it can be adapted to the patient's changes in motor skills as the disease advances. The program also needs to remain challenging to the patient so it's effective, but safety is also paramount.

Dr Colleen Canning says some people find that their tremor gets worse during exercise, but their symptoms improve post-training. Others will experience a significant level of anxiety because they feel overwhelmed.

> *If people are doing moderate to high intensity exercise,*
> *which makes them puff, I would recommend [exercise] be*
> *done when their medication is working optimally.*
> —Dr Colleen Canning

Professor Meg Morris says a vigorous exercise program can suit the needs of some people. Others might prefer alternative exercise solutions. There is no single recipe for exercise that suits everyone. That's because the disease is so individual and manifests in different ways. It's important for people with Parkinson's to have their own plan to optimise movement, with advice from a skilled professional.

Dr Canning says people who have an established exercise routine before diagnosis generally continue with their good habits. But people who don't have a history of regular exercise should seek professional help before embarking on a program.

*One of the biggest challenges is getting the person to perform
effective exercise that is safe.*

—Dr Colleen Canning

Cost can be a major obstacle when it comes to starting an exercise program that is both challenging and safe. One-on-one supervision can be expensive and often involves a home visit from a physiotherapist. Some private health insurance policies cover the cost and government assistance benefits will depend on individual circumstances.

Dr Canning would like to see special areas set up in community centres to cater for people with disabilities, offering such things as trained assistance to help people get on and off machines. And in an ideal world, subsidised transport would enable people to get there and return home.

'None of us find it entertaining to exercise at home over long periods of time. For some people with Parkinson's disease, if they don't exercise at home there are no facilities or funding to do anything else,' Dr Canning says.

Neurologist Dr Scott Whyte says some people think they can only exercise in the gym or when using a piece of equipment such as an exercise bike. But, he says: 'There are forms of exercise for everyone even for people who are confined to a chair in institutional care'. Simply moving in and out of a chair can also help with fitness.

When exercising at home, carers can help supervise but they are often dealing with competing demands. Carers themselves also need to keep up with their own activities and to maintain their fitness.

What the patients say

Nerissa Mapes, aged 33, found yoga confronting, because she was forced to use her fine motor skills and balancing became difficult. She said doing a yoga class reduced her to tears.

'It reminded me I couldn't do certain things and certain moves. So I ended up doing one-on-one sessions with the yoga instructor.'

Nerissa's Parkinson's medication made her lose a significant amount of weight. She felt weak and started working out with a personal trainer at the gym. After 15 minutes she felt exhausted, but after several weeks exercising made her feel much better. She says she prefers doing weights at the gym rather than having to face yoga classes.

> *Having the strength in my body, made me feel mentally stronger.*
> —Nerissa Mapes, diagnosed in her 20s

Nerissa also believes massage helped to loosen her joints. 'My body's very rigid and stiff. It feels like being wrapped in wire most of the time. Massage can be good, but I don't have it done regularly.'

Paula Argy, aged 39, keeps fit by walking along the beach. She also tried Bikram yoga for four years, which requires exercising in a heated room. 'The only reason why I stopped was because of the heat,' she said. But she found it very useful. 'It strengthened a lot of my core and my muscles,' Paula said. She believes practising yoga prevented her from falling, which is one of her biggest fears. 'That's why I don't live on my own with my kids. I live with my parents now. I worry that if I fall my kids will be there, and I just can't have that happen.'

Exercise of any form is good, there is no question about that,' says 73-year-old John Silk. He believes it delays the setbacks that come with the disease. John says he enjoyed hydrotherapy and playing golf, but now sticks to weekly personal training sessions that target balance and keeping his upper torso strong. He has been taught exercises that help him get out of bed and walk down the corridor without losing balance. 'They're all specifically Parkinson's orientated,' he says.

Neil Sligar's story

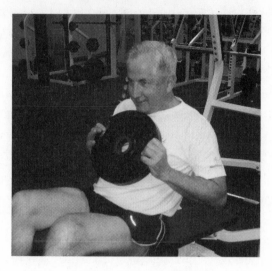

Neil Sligar is a Sydney financial planner who advocates vigorous exercise.

I was diagnosed with Parkinson's disease in 1998. Developing the illness was beyond my control, whereas potentially worse conditions such as heart attack and stroke were largely within my control through changing from a sedentary lifestyle. I've adopted a program at the gym which is aimed at improving flexibility, pushing heart and lungs (endurance), and increasing strength.

In the year 2000, my physical capacity probably differed little from many other 54-year-old men. Nowadays, at 63, my physical performance is ahead of what it was nine years ago.

I attend a gym three or four times a week. A typical session comprises:

- 5–10 minutes of stretching
- 10–15 minutes aerobic activity, such as cycling
- 35–40 minutes weightlifting, focusing on different parts of my body.

I find that the harder my session, the more relaxed and relieved of Parkinson's I feel for the next few hours. My tremor sometimes increases immediately following exertion but soon subsides.

In February 2008 I competed in the Aquafit Gym's Summer Iron Man Challenge. In February 2009, I bench-pressed 110 kilograms at a body weight of around 86 kilograms.

How has Parkinson's disease impacted my training?

Very little. My treadmill running is poor due to dragging of my right leg and there's rigidity in my right arm as fatigue sets in. On the bike, I feel unhindered by Parkinson's disease. In weightlifting, my 'explosive' capability is diminished. For example, snapping weights on a bar to my shoulders is significantly impeded.

The importance of a little puffing for those of us with Parkinson's disease is recognised by an increasing number of professionals. This has been described by Dr Michael Okun in his article 'What's hot in Parkinson's disease' on the National Parkinson's Foundation website.

My training routine is not tailored as Parkinson's therapy. I do it for general health, because I enjoy it, and because setting targets provides a constant challenge.

Outside the gym, in the office, supermarket and post office, my tremor and awkwardness are obvious as the effect of medication wanes. People are kind and understanding, although when they offer to carry my briefcase or shopping bags I politely decline.

I absorb advice from people whose wisdom I respect. My progress has benefited from the generosity of those who've guided me. Many fitness instructors have gone out of their way to help, with their tips and encouragement.

One thing at a time

Sometimes people with Parkinson's disease have trouble doing two things at a time. Movements performed without much concentration (automatic movements) are affected more than movements that require concentration and direction. When we perform two things at the same time, our concentration on each task is reduced, and people with Parkinson's disease are more likely to experience freezing or impaired movements.

Common problems include difficulties in talking while walking, eating or driving. Another problem can be walking while carrying objects.

> *You can't do two things at once. When I go shopping because I'm looking for something, I make sure I don't lose my handbag. I'm checking prices, and making sure the steps are right. By the time I get to the cash register I stop thinking. You look like you've got a mental health problem. I find that very frustrating.*
> —Karen Rowland, diagnosed in her 40s

> *I get a foggy brain, where I can't think clearly. My brain kind of stops basically. If you understand what's going on, it makes it so much easier to deal with. You're not going mad. It will pass and you'll get through it.*
> —Paula Argy, young mother with Parkinson's

Professor Meg Morris says people can use a number of strategies to avoid the problem, especially when their safety is at risk. For example, if you're walking along the road, talking on the phone can be dangerous, and you are more likely to fall. A Parkinson's patient should focus on their footsteps and taking long strides so they move safely.

> *If there's a critical need to maintain safety, or do a particular task well, then it's best to do one thing at a time ... and to relax.*
> —Professor Meg Morris

Professor Morris outlines a range of strategies in her book *Moving Ahead with Parkinson's*.[9] Here are some of her suggestions.

- Break up long movement sequences into separate steps, and do only one movement in the sequence at a time. For example, when getting out of bed, rather than rolling over like a log, break it down into steps. Turn the head, shoulders, knees, and legs over before sitting up.
- Avoid doing two things at once, such as carrying a tray of drinks when walking, or talking when writing.
- Consciously think about each movement before doing it. Rehearse it mentally before starting to move.
- Carefully attend to each movement while doing it.
- Use cues to trigger a movement: for example, visual cues (cards, adhesive tape on the floor), auditory cues (key words, short phrases, music) and movement cues (rocking from side to side).
- Arrange the home environment to make it easier to move around and reduce the chances of falling.

Table 5.1 also gives some suggestions on managing some everyday activities safely. Not everyone will need to use these strategies, and a person in the early stages might be more than capable of multi-tasking.

One of the challenges is to work out who will benefit most from the techniques. Dr Colleen Canning says if a person notices that when they start talking, their walking deteriorates, then they should be given instructions to help. 'I don't believe one size fits all. Some people are capable of working things out for themselves ... others need guidance.'

Table 5.1 Managing everyday activities safely

Common activity	Suggestions
Going for a walk with a friend	Concentrate primarily on your walking. If you want to maintain a conversation, stop every so often to talk. Do not try to walk and talk at the same time.
Walking and carrying objects	Use a bag or trolley so you can concentrate on walking.
Walking to and from the shower with your clothes	Dress and undress in your bedroom, and wear a dressing gown while walking between rooms.
Carrying medication from the kitchen to dining room	Use a small trolley or mobile tray.
Paying for shopping	Wait for or ask for the total payment before you reach for your money. Have the money you will need for a particular shopping trip, such as a weekly supermarket trip, in a separate purse.
Driving with a passenger	Avoid driving and talking. Pull over if you need to talk.
At the dinner table	If you want to have a conversation, choose times during the meal to pause from eating to speak or listen.

Adapted from Morris, Iansek and Kirkwood, *Moving Ahead with Parkinson's*, Buscombe Vicprint Ltd, Victoria

Finding help

Physiotherapists who have experience in prescribing exercise programs for people with Parkinson's disease can be found in two main ways. Patients can get a referral from their local doctor to a physiotherapy rehabilitation outpatients department at a public hospital. You should check that the department caters for people who have neurological conditions. Patients can also contact the Australian Physiotherapy Association at www.physiotherapy.asn.au and click on the red 'Find a Physio' button on the right of the screen. Ask for the contact details of physiotherapists in your local area who have an interest in neurology or aged care (gerontology).

Speech problems

The impact [problems with speech] has on someone's daily life and relationships is immeasurable. We take for granted the ability to communicate and swallow, until something goes wrong.

—Melanie Tewman, speech pathologist

Communication forms a big part of our daily life, enabling us to perform everyday tasks, while maintaining and building relationships. Speech is something many of us take for granted. It's a relatively simple function, like breathing.

Up to 75 per cent of people living with Parkinson's disease experience communication changes. Most of them report problems during the middle to advanced stages of the disease. This can have a huge impact on people psychologically, creating feelings of frustration and resulting in them withdrawing from social circles.

Speech problems can manifest in various ways. Speech pathologist Melanie Tewman says voice projection is a common issue. People who have Parkinson's disease tend to start speaking more softly, and others struggle to hear what they're saying. Patients are often asked to repeat themselves when their speech is affected in this way, and communication becomes frustrating and difficult.

> *The ability to speak at a 'normal' volume becomes difficult to do automatically.*
>
> —Melanie Tewman

The quality of the voice can also change: it can become hoarse and more monotone. Articulation can become difficult, resulting in a slurring or mumbling of words. Speech pathologist Anne Beirne says the quality of articulation can deteriorate because of poor muscle control and co-ordination. 'We find that the smaller muscles will reduce the function of speech and swallowing. A person's words tend to run together and become less distinct.' Anne Beirne also says:

> *Language can also be affected, and a person might struggle to retrieve words and put them in a structured format. Specific language problems can include word finding, and difficulties with starting and following conversations.*
>
> *These communication issues can be enormously frustrating—particularly for people who were functioning very well in their previous world. They tend to struggle expressing their opinions. People who were once the life of a party will find it harder to keep up with punchy responses. It can be very distressing and cause significant social withdrawal. People sometimes make a conscious decision not to socialise because they find it too stressful.*

Anne says varying the dose of Parkinson's medications may reduce the problem. But the benefit may depend on a person's 'on' and 'off' periods. 'If their medication is working well, their problems might not be as great,' she says.

> *About three-quarters of people with Parkinson's will at some point experience communication change. Initially it might be quite subtle, and in the early stages people will find they're able to mask their communication issues.*
>
> —Melanie Tewman

> *My voice is very soft. You can't get anyone's attention and it makes you feel invisible in the world sometimes.*
>
> —Nerissa Mapes, diagnosed in her 20s

Types of speech problems

The most common speech problems for Parkinson's disease patients are:

- Voice projection is reduced.
- A soft, husky voice develops, which is difficult for others to hear.
- Reduced fluency or rhythm of speech ('stuttering like') may develop.
- The melody and intonation of speech change.
- Articulation and clarity of speech sounds ('slurring', 'mumbling') are reduced.
- Patients may experience difficulties in thinking of words and getting out what they want to say in a timely manner.[10]

Managing speech problems

Many speech pathologists in Australia use the Lee Silverman Voice Treatment (LSVT) program, an accredited program that was developed in the United States. In this treatment, patients are taught a series of exercises to improve vocal intensity and quality. The program also teaches patients to become aware of the effort required to produce the level of voice volume they need, so they can correct themselves. There are some mantras like 'think loud, think of shouting'. The treatment is intensive and a person is usually required to participate in 16 sessions with a speech pathologist over a month.

Anne Beirne says this program is highly effective. 'It's very powerful and people normally get results straight away.'

> *It focuses on one particular technique rather than bamboozling the patient with a number of things to improve their communication. In Parkinson's disease, multi-tasking is a huge problem so we really need to keep the strategies very simple and clear.*

A patient needs to completely redefine what level of effort is required to produce a normal-sounding voice. The repetiveness and intensity of the program is important for this behavioural change.

A study of the effects of Lee Silverman Voice Treatment on swallowing and voice in eight patients who had Parkinson's disease was published in 2002. The program achieved a 51 per cent reduction in the number of swallowing disorders in the group. There was also a significant increase in vocal intensity.

The book *Moving Ahead with Parkinson's*, which Professor Meg Morris co-authored, also proposes the following strategies for improving speech for Parkinson's patients.

- Think carefully about what you are going to say before starting to say it.
- Break up the message into short phrases, for example, 'I'll talk to you ... about the matter ... when I get home.'
- Break up longer words into syllables, for example: 'u/ni/ver/si/ty'.

- Take a breath before each group of phrases, as this will help you speak louder.
- We speak on expired air, so keep air 'flowing' throughout the phrase. Patients are generally encouraged to take a big breath before speaking and to talk while exhaling. If expired air is running out, stop and take another big breath before speaking. Practising breathing techniques will encourage better, louder voice production.
- Further, if your voice is soft, imagine the listener is farther away and think about speaking louder to reach them.

Parkinson's disease can affect a person's facial expressions because the size and speed of muscles controlling facial movement are reduced. People who are affected, struggle with being outwardly expressive and their face becomes mask-like in appearance. In the early stages, facial expression may be affected only slightly and then worsen over time. It can cause social problems because the lack of spontaneous expression may lead people to think that the person with Parkinson's is disinterested or sad. Speech pathology can help people become more aware of the problem so they can consciously control facial movements. Specific exercises are used to help facial muscles move more freely. In 2003, a study examined the effects of Lee Silverman's Voice Treatment on facial expression. Forty-four patients took part in the study, which showed that intensive voice therapy improved a person's expression (voice, face and gesture).

Swallowing problems

About 50 per cent of people living with Parkinson's disease experience swallowing difficulties (dysphagia). Problems can range from mild to severe. Speech pathologist Anne Beirne says swallowing problems don't necessarily evolve at the same rate as movement problems.

Some people with quite advanced motor problems might
still have a reasonably intact swallow. The biggest concern,
from a medical point of view, is the risk of aspiration of food
and fluid getting into the airways, causing lung infection.
Aspiration pneumonia is a common cause of death among
people with Parkinson's disease. This type of pneumonia
is caused by something 'foreign' entering the airways and
causing infection. It can be caused by food, fluid, saliva or a
person's vomit.

Swallowing is a highly complex neurological manoeuvre.
It takes 26 different sets of muscles to perform one swallow.
And it takes half the nerves coming off the brain to activate
those muscles.

—Melanie Tewman

There are several warning signs that someone is developing swallowing problems. A significant sign is coughing while eating or drinking, because this indicates that food is getting into the airway. Prolonged chewing or avoiding certain foods, such as steak, because they are more difficult to swallow are other signs.

People who have very dry mouths and throats, even without reduced muscle function, may also experience swallowing difficulties.

Swallowing problems, like speech problems, can lead to social isolation because a person may feel they cannot eat or drink like others. Anne Beirne says they affect people's ability to socialise. 'They become very self-conscious about their eating behaviour in public so they'll often withdraw from social situations.'

Swallowing problems can interfere with medication if tablets become harder to swallow or get lodged in the throat.

Types of swallowing problems

- Half the people with Parkinson's disease are affected by swallowing problems.

- Problems can occur with food, fluids, medications or saliva.
- Swallowing problems can lead to choking, pneumonia, dehydration and malnutrition.
- Coughing when eating or drinking is an early sign of developing problems with swallowing.[11]

Saliva problems can affect up to 75 per cent of people with Parkinson's disease, as a result of changes in swallowing, the effects of medication or for other reasons, such as an altered diet or as a direct effect of the disease. Saliva problems can lead to a dry mouth, drooling or thick saliva that is difficult to clear.

Speech pathologist Anne Beirne says:

Sometimes people can experience problems with both excess saliva and oral dryness. We believe the latter is linked to Parkinson's disease medication. Excess saliva is most likely the result of reduced frequency of automatic swallowing, which clears saliva.

People feel very uncomfortable when they're seen to be dribbling. Their clothes can become soiled, speech can be a problem and it can make it very difficult to go out and do things. Caregivers can also become very stressed and embarrassed about it. The problem usually affects people in the middle to advanced stages of the disease. Some people in the early stages may report dampness on their pillows overnight because of their weak mouth posture.

Managing swallowing problems

There are no strategies available to reverse swallowing problems. Instead, someone who has swallowing difficulties can use strategies to compensate for the loss by paying more attention to their eating habits. Sitting upright while eating and drinking, taking smaller bites of food, and avoiding any distractions while eating can help. A simple strategy like 'swallow before you speak' can make a big difference in social situations. Anne Beirne says swallowing problems can become worse if a person rushes while eating. Eating more slowly and carefully is generally the rule for people with issues. Patients can seek guidance from a speech pathologist to develop the right strategies for each individual.

Moving Ahead with Parkinson's suggests the following strategies for helping to manage swallowing difficulties:

- Consciously think about swallowing as you do it.
- Do one task at a time. For example, avoid reaching for an object or talking while swallowing.
- To help with swallowing, try reading a cue card that says '1, 2, 3, swallow'.
- Before you swallow, make sure that the food is in the middle of the tongue.
- Using a mirror can help place food or medication on the centre of the tongue.
- Make sure the lips are closed when you are trying to swallow.
- Take one sip of liquid at a time.
- Place your hand on your Adam's apple to ensure that you complete each swallow before starting the next one.
- Ask people to give you time to finish swallowing before they ask you questions or get you to join in a conversation.

If swallowing problems are more advanced, a patient might need to make changes to their diet so food and liquids can be swallowed more easily. This is often recommended when there are clear clinical signs that the patient is at risk of inhaling fluids into their lungs. The signs include coughing, straining the voice, making a gurgling sound and if the person chokes after swallowing. A speech pathologist will assess the patient and make appropriate recommendations such as making dietary changes. Drinking denser fluids slows the process of swallowing which will reduce the risk of fluids going down the wrong way (the lungs). Fluids can be thickened by adding a recommended powder which is colourless, odourless and tasteless. Levels of thickness can vary from mildly thick (similar to gravy) to moderately thick (like a thick shake). According to Anne Beirne, in cases of severe swallowing difficulties, the patient may require fluids to be pudding thick (the consistency of mousse). A speech pathologist will provide patients and their caregivers with all the information needed to thicken fluids so the problem can be managed easily in the home.

If food can't be tolerated, changing its consistency will also make eating easier. For example, cooking food for a bit longer, adding sauce to make it moister or mashing the ingredients may help prevent choking. Anne Beirne says any food can be pureed to a lump-free consistency by using a handheld mixer or blender. 'Again, the recommendation to have foods pureed would be made following a formal assessment, and if the patient was having extreme difficulty chewing or swallowing unmodified foods.' There are other ways to address the problem in less severe cases. Soft moist foods are recommended for minor problems, or minced foods for moderately severe swallowing difficulties. Most foods can be cooked and prepared to the recommended consistency and patients are usually able to have a normal diet (range of foods) with only some exclusions: when foods remain tough, dry and/or crumbly despite extended cooking, mincing or blending.

When a patient experiences extreme swallowing difficulties and is not receiving adequate nutrition or hydration orally, then other methods are recommended. PEG feeding will prevent someone from becoming malnourished. PEG stands for percutaneous endoscopic gastrostomy (also known as enteral feeding by gastrostomy). This is where an opening is made in the stomach so a permanent feeding tube can be inserted. A specially prepared liquid-based food is injected into this tube and deposited directly into the stomach. A dietitian will prescribe this liquid food and suggest the frequency of feeding. Anne Beirne says full nutritional and hydration requirements can be maintained exclusively using a PEG. 'In some instances, where the patient can tolerate small amounts of food/fluid safely, they may have a combination of PEG feeding with oral intake for comfort and quality of life purposes.'

Looking after your diet

The most important dietary advice for a person living with Parkinson's disease is to eat a healthy, balanced diet. While most people find they lose weight, others might put on extra kilos because movement problems affect their ability to exercise. Advice from an expert will ensure a person's dietary needs are met, while getting the most out of their medications by adjusting meal times.

Weight loss

Weight loss is a common problem for people with Parkinson's disease. There are multiple reasons and some are not clearly defined. It's thought that for Parkinson's patients the body's metabolic rate is faster and energy burn is more significant when movements increase. Swallowing difficulties (dysphagia) and other related issues can also compromise nutrition and hydration. Clinical experience shows that unintentional weight loss can occur even when there are no apparent changes to eating habits.[12] Dietitian Alison Stewart says periodic weight loss, constipation[13] and the increased risk of food interfering with medications, usually occur in the middle to later stages of disease.

Nerissa Mapes says she lost weight after her medications caused nausea. 'One woman asked whether I lost the weight on purpose, and I said, actually no, I need help.' Nerissa said anti-nausea tablets helped relieve the side effects of her Parkinson's medications.

Drug interactions

In Parkinson's disease, the rate at which the stomach empties can be slower. If medications are taken with meals, there could be a delay in absorption compared with when they're taken on an empty stomach. This delay in the effects of the medication can be a big issue for people in the middle to late stages of the illness, because they rely more heavily on levodopa to control their symptoms.

In general, Alison Stewart says it's best to separate your meals and Parkinson's medications so that pills are taken at least 30–45 minutes before eating. Adjusting the amount of foods containing protein and other nutrients may also help, although it's also important to eat protein because it's necessary for good health. Alison Stewart also recommends getting individual advice from a specialist dietitian to ensure optimal and predictable action from Parkinson's medications.

Dr Michael Hayes, neurologist, says a small number of patients who take levodopa have severe motor fluctuations because their high-protein diet interferes with the drug. This effect can be more profound in the later stages of disease.

In the mid to late 1980s, patients were often advised to avoid protein-rich foods during the day so they didn't reduce the effect of levodopa. These foods include meat, chicken, fish, nuts, legumes and dairy products. However, this advice caused other nutrient deficiencies and a worsening of Parkinson's symptoms at night.

More recently, research has focused on spreading protein intake throughout the day and increasing the amount of carbohydrates during each meal and snack.[14] Carbohydrate foods include breads, cereals, fruits and vegetables. Preliminary results suggest that less 'off' time from their medication can be achieved by including more carbohydrates at each meal and snack, while maintaining an adequate protein intake for a healthy diet. See the general nutrition guidelines below for more on foods and good health.

Dietitian Alison Stewart says manipulating a dietary plan, and particularly the timing of meals 30–45 minutes after medications, can potentially improve the control of symptoms for people with Parkinson's by providing a more predictable response to levodopa therapy.

Experience suggests that increasing the carbohydrate-to-protein ratio in the diet is a useful therapy in later stages for treating weight loss, and to lessen the effect of protein interference with medication. However, a high-carbohydrate diet aimed at treating weight loss may not be ideal for people who also suffer from diabetes or are overweight or obese.

Strategies for managing diet problems

Certain foods, vitamins or unusual diets are sometimes claimed to relieve Parkinson's disease symptoms, but there is no evidence to support these claims.

One common story is that broad beans (fava beans) help treat Parkinson's disease. Although broad beans contain levodopa, it is only in variable and small amounts, and nowhere near the level found in medications. The number of beans you would have to eat for them to have an effect would probably make you ill in other ways.

Patients tempted by any unusual dietary therapies should seek medical guidance. Your doctor/specialist, a registered dietitian, occupational therapist, speech pathologist or Parkinson's disease nurse may be able to advise on diet and practical issues with eating.[15]

Good nutrition involves eating the right amount of carbo-hydrates, proteins, fat, vitamins and minerals. While the levels required vary according to individual needs, it is important for everyone to eat a varied and well-balanced diet.

A good guide to healthy eating is to choose from each of the food groups. The minimum number of serves recommended per day for each food group is listed below. The actual require-ments vary with age, sex, body size and your activity level. A balanced diet should contain a combination of all the nutrients needed to keep the body healthy and in good repair.[16]

Remember—variety within each food group is important!

Meats and their alternatives: 1 serve (or 2 small serves)
- Source of protein and other nutrients, e.g. iron, zinc and vitamin B12.
- Regular intake of oily fish, such as tuna, salmon, mack-erel, perch, sardines and herring are good sources of Omega-3 fatty acids, which are recommended for gen-eral health.
- Sample serve is 100g of lean beef, lamb, pork, chicken, fish or two eggs or two-thirds of a cup of cooked legumes.

Milk and milk products: 3–4 serves
- Source of protein, calcium and other micronutrients.
- Sample serve is 250ml milk/custard or 40g of cheese or 200g tub of yoghurt.

Fruit: 2 serves
- Source of carbohydrate, dietary fibre and micronutrients, e.g. folate, vitamins C and A and other micronutrients.
- Sample serve is 1 piece of medium-sized fruit (i.e. apple) or 2 pieces of smaller sized fruit (i.e. apricots).
- 1 cup fruit salad/canned fruit or one-third of a cup of dried fruit or 120ml fruit juice.

Vegetables: 5 serves
- Source of carbohydrate, dietary fibre and micronutrients, e.g. folate, vitamins C and A and other micronutrients.
- Sample serve of vegetables is 1 medium potato or ½ cup cooked vegetables, peas, beans or lentils or 1 cup of salad vegetables.

Breads and cereals: 5+ serves
- Source of carbohydrate, dietary fibre, vitamin B and other micronutrients.
- 1 serve is equal to 1 slice of bread or ½ large bread roll or ½ cup of cooked pasta/rice or $^2/_3$ cup of cereal.

Fluids: at least 6–8 glasses (200ml glass)
- Important for adequate hydration.
- Fluids can include water, juices, cordial, milk, tea, coffee, soup.

When taken in an adequate diet, micronutrients (vitamins and minerals) will help to avoid the need for supplements. Vitamins A, D, E and K are fat-soluble, and remain in the body for weeks before being depleted. Vitamin A helps with maintaining healthy eyesight, skin and teeth. It's also good for the reproductive system. It can be found in milk, cheese, eggs, fatty fish, yellow-orange vegetables and fruits, such as carrots, pumpkin, mango and apricots, and other vegetables, such as spinach and broccoli. The main source of vitamin D is produced by the action of sunlight on the skin. Diet is not the main source of vitamin D, although it's found in some foods such as fortified margarine, salmon, herring, mackerel and eggs. Major sources of vitamin E include nuts and seeds, seed oil, spinach and fish. Vitamin K is predominantly found in green leafy vegetables and, to a lesser extent, dairy foods; they include spinach, salad greens, cabbage, broccoli, brussel sprouts, soybean oil, canola oil and margarines.[17]

If there's a need to supplement the diet with fat-soluble vitamins, only take in amounts that match the recommended dietary intake dose or what's advised by your dietitian or doctor. This is due to the potentially toxic effects of taking high doses of some fat-soluble vitamins.

B complex vitamins and vitamin C are water soluble and need to be replenished daily. B vitamins are found in bread and cereals, while vitamin C is mostly found in fruits and vegetables. Citrus fruits such as oranges are particularly good sources.

Minerals are found in many foods. Some of the important minerals are calcium, iron, zinc and magnesium.

Neurologist Dr Scott Whyte says low bone calcium levels are common in people with Parkinson's disease, and this may be associated with increased fracture risk in the event of a fall. Adequate calcium and vitamin D intake are important, as well as regular exercise and sunlight exposure (indirect sunlight exposure is adequate). He says an assessment of bone mineral density may be useful, as medication might be required when bone densities are too low. Your general practitioner may help you in this regard.

Dietitian Alison Stewart provides a list of common dietary issues that people who have Parkinson's disease face, and the strategies that can be used to address them. She says if weight loss is an issue, it's best to increase energy intake by either eating more or by fortifying your diet with extra carbohydrate. These include wholemeal breads, cereals, fruit, some vegetables and foods containing healthy fats such as polyunsaturated or monounsaturated margarines, oils and avocado. Protein should not be increased beyond the recommended dietary levels unless specifically advised to, due to the risk of interference with Parkinson's medications. A dietitian can help make changes to suit an individual's lifestyle and usual eating patterns.

If constipation becomes a problem, Alison Stewart says it's

best to eat a diet high in fibre (wholemeal breads, cereals, fruit and vegetables) and to drink plenty of fluids, at least six to eight 200ml glasses a day. Pears, prunes and the juice from these fruits have natural laxative properties and can be useful additions to your diet. If constipation persists, then a doctor can recommend laxatives.

Table 5.2 Some strategies for dealing with dietary problems

Problem	Management strategies
Loss of body weight and poor nutritional status because of increased energy needs and/or reduced food intake, which may affect medication	Increase energy and nutrient intake with energy-dense foods and fluids such as carbohydrates or healthy fat containing foods. See below for examples Consume protein-containing foods up to recommended dietary amounts only. Amounts higher than this are more likely to cause an interference with the action of the medication in mid to late stage Parkinson's disease Address swallowing problems, constipation, fatigue and dental health. See below
Eating and swallowing problems	Get a speech pathology assessment for safe swallowing strategies and advice on changes to food and fluid textures necessary for a safe swallow. Then seek a dietitian's advice on a texture-modified diet that will meet your individual nutrition and hydration needs. A texture modified diet is one where the food is made softer, minced or pureed for ease of chewing and swallowing. Sometimes advice may be given for using thickened fluids. Fluids can be thickened using special formulas

Fatigue and eating food slowly	Choose smaller, higher energy, denser meals, snacks and supplements which are not too high in protein. Some snack examples include: 1 slice of raisin toast with polyunsaturated/ monounsaturated/canola based margarine; ½ cup flavoured milk drink, plus a banana a fruit scone with margarine and jam a tub (200g) fruit yoghurt with 1 tablespoon mixed dried fruit and 1 cup fruit juice a cup of thick vegetable soup; 4 water cracker biscuits + margarine + ½ thin slice cheese + tomato + 1 cup fruit juice Only use higher protein supplements under direction of a specialist dietitian Choose times for eating and drinking at times when fatigue is likely to be reduced
Interference of diet with the action of medication (levodopa)	Consider a medical review of dosage and timing For optimal results, take medications on an empty stomach, at least 30-45 minutes before meals and snacks; if nausea is a problem, eat a small snack containing carbohydrate, such as a biscuit or pureed fruit with medications Consume protein-containing foods up to recommended dietary amounts only. Amounts higher than this are more likely to cause an interference with the action of medication in the mid to later stage of Parkinson's disease. Consult a dietitian for advice on diet to reduce the risk of interference with drugs (for instance, as to whether a patient needs a diet higher in carbohydrate relative to protein)

Constipation (this can be severe and needs special attention)	Consume a high-fibre diet by eating wholemeal breads and cereals, fruits and vegetables. Seek advice from a doctor or dietitian on laxative therapy if diet alone does not resolve the issue
Dry mouth, poor dental health and thick saliva	See your dentist regularly Sip water regularly, including during meals Eat moist foods with gravies or sauces added Moisten your mouth and throat before swallowing medications Check that your fluid intake is adequate Eat sugar-free sweets or suck on ice blocks between meals Try chewing sugarless gum Use a vaporiser/humidifier at night Use a steam vapour inhaler e.g. Bosistos Ensure regular tooth brushing and dental flossing Use Biotene toothpaste (available from your chemist) Use a mouth wash e.g. Chlorhexidine or Biotene Limit alcohol as this makes a dry mouth worse Get advice on saliva management from a speech pathologist

Adapted from Alison Stewart (2008), 'Nutrition: The Parkinson's diet', *Australian Ageing Agenda*, January/February, p 66. Reproduced with permission.

Where to get dietary advice

People who want to learn more about diet strategies will find the following sources useful.

1. Individual consultation with a dietitian at clinics specialising in movement disorders. Dietitians may be found at your local community health centre, medical centre or they may work in private practice.
2. Find an accredited practising dietitian from the Dietitians Association of Australia website: www.daa.asn.au
3. The publication *Eating Well, Stay Well with Parkinson's disease* is available from Parkinson's Australia in your state or territory.
4. www.nutritioncanlivewith.com is the website of US dietitian Kathrynne Holden, who specialises in Parkinson's disease.
5. General information on nutrition can be found be at: the Dietitians Association of Australian website, www.daa.asn.au, go to the link 'Smart Eating for You'; Nutrition Australia website: www.nutritionaustralia.org; and. Parkinson's Victoria website: www.parkinsonsvic.org.au.
6. Bone Health: Osteoporosis Australia website: http//osteoporosis.org.au for articles on vitamin D, calcium and safe access to sunlight.

Managing at home

> We don't want people to quit if they find [things] difficult. We encourage them to plan their day and live life to the full. They can't win against Parkinson's disease because it's a progressive illness, but they can still plan their day and tell the disease 'this is my time now, I can enjoy it.'
> —Margarita Makoutonina, occupational therapist

If a person is having trouble walking around the home or completing simple tasks, then occupational therapists and physiotherapists can provide valuable advice. Home visits are often needed so they can assess whether changes are necessary.

Occupational therapist Margarita Makoutonina says it's best to keep the home uncluttered to avoid creating hazards and make it easier for someone with Parkinson's to move around safely. She says 'we look at the layout of the house and if a person has problems with mobility, we may need to relocate the furniture', to keep the environment open. Light and bright colours, and white also help the brain function more effectively.

Therapists also teach practical strategies to help patients overcome problems, such as getting off a chair or out of bed. Generally, practical techniques are used before aids or technology are introduced in the home. 'We try not to introduce equipment or technology straight away. If we do, [patients are] not using their muscles properly. As the saying goes, use it or lose it,' says Margarita Makoutonina.

Strategies for managing at home[18]

Bedroom

Turning in bed can be a problem for people at any stage of their disease, even in the early years. The best way to manage this is to bend the knees, face the direction you want to turn and reach across with the opposite arm. Satin bed sheets are useful to help slide the body. Margarita Makoutonina says it's cheaper to use satin nightwear or a piece of silky material about 1 metre wide, which can be placed across the bed and tucked under the mattress or stitched onto the existing sheet.

Bathroom

A stool in the shower and grab rails in the alcove or on the bath will help people manage their balance. A handheld shower hose and long-handled bath sponge are also helpful. Sometimes a shower screen needs to be replaced for safety reasons in case someone loses their balance. Husband and carer Dan Mongan says he spent about $300 to replace a glass screen with curtains, and to install hand bars in the shower recess, toilet and backyard. Using a chair to sit on while cleaning teeth may make the process easier (regular dental check-ups are also a good idea).

Toilet

Handrails beside the toilet can improve safety. Fixed and portable aids are available to raise the height of toilet seats. Bedside commodes will avoid the need to walk to the toilet during the night, or non-spill urinals and bedpans can be placed near the bed.

Dressing

It's recommended that people retrain their fine motor skills rather than change their wardrobe. For example, it's best to sit down while changing clothes or doing up buttons. Maintaining balance takes up a lot of energy, so sitting down allows the mind to be completely devoted to the job at hand. To focus on doing one thing at a time, it's best not to talk to anyone while dressing. Button hooks can help do up buttons if other practical techniques fail. Velcro is easier to manage at the bottom of a buttoned shirt. Clothing that has elastic waistbands or is made from stretch fabric is easy to manage. Leather-soled shoes provide less friction than rubber to make walking easier.

> *Dressing's hard. I wear a lot of gym gear because it's easier to get on and off. Buttons are out.*
> —Paula Argy, young mother with Parkinson's disease

Telephones

For patients experiencing hand tremor, telephones with big buttons are easier to use. Having an answering machine turned on at all times avoids having to rush to the phone—occupational therapist Margarita Makoutonina says rushing to answer a call often leads to anxiety and stress, and the person tends to freeze. 'To overcome this, we encourage patients to do one thing at a time,' she says. They should set up the phone, pen and writing pad on a table by a chair, which should be positioned somewhere in an open space so they can be reached easily. It's often very difficult for people with Parkinson's disease to do other things while talking on the phone.

Reading and writing

Bookstands can be used while reading in bed or in the living room, and both manual or automated page turners are available. When writing, warm up the hands by drawing large loops. Pens with larger grips give more control. Lined paper helps maintain the size of the writing. If handwriting becomes illegible, switch to using a computer. A key guard on a keyboard helps ensure the correct key is pressed.

> I want to have a long and successful career in communications. I really enjoy what I do. But typing can sometimes be difficult. It's the tool of the trade, so down the track I might have to get voice recognition software. I'll see what happens.
>
> —Nerissa Mapes, diagnosed in her 20s

Medication management

> When they're at home, or at work and busy doing something or multi-tasking, they [patients] often forget about their medication or delay them ... and get into trouble.
>
> —Margarita Makoutonina

One way to manage medication and ensure the right pills are taken at the right time is to use a pill box. A range of boxes is available to remind patients when to take medication. Dosage containers are available for daily or weekly organisation of pills. A timing device that reminds you when to take your medication will give peace of mind. Devices that can be used include watches (with several alarms), kitchen clocks and computers. Mobile phones are okay, but current models are too complicated to operate and require intact fine motor skills, which is a problem for many people. (If your medication regime is the same each day, then someone else may be able to program your mobile phone for you.) Pill cutters and tablet crushers are handy for measuring the correct dose.

Sleeping problems

Most people with Parkinson's disease suffer from poor sleep and this affects their ability to function properly the following day.

Sleep disturbance isn't confined only to the evening. If people have a poor night's sleep, then the effects can spill into the daytime. Occupational therapist Margarita Makoutonina says if people don't get a proper rest their symptoms are exacerbated. They can become emotional and the effect of medication is diminished, which means symptoms are not well controlled. Some dopamine agonists and levodopa can induce sleepiness in people with Parkinson's. Anyone who experiences a sudden desire to sleep during the day should be warned about doing activities that can compromise safety, such as driving and operating machinery.

Ms Makoutonina says people can use various techniques to prevent themselves from sleeping during the day. Rearranging their routine, for instance, will help them keep active and stimulated. A relaxation session might be required during the day. All this can be organised with the help of an occupational therapist to take into account the individual's abilities, needs and wants. 'If we don't have enough sleep during night-time, it affects us during the day. Part of my role is to make the patient aware of day sleep,' says Ms Makoutonina.

Possible causes of poor sleep[19]

There are a host of reasons why people can't sleep properly at night, perhaps attributable to the disease itself or to a side effect of medications.

Drugs wear off

When levodopa or other dopamine replacement drugs start to wear off or lose their effectiveness, common Parkinson's symptoms start to take hold. These include stiffness, tremor, pain and problems moving or turning in bed. If these symptoms develop during sleep, they disturb the sleep cycle.

Early morning dystonia

Sleep can also be disrupted if a person experiences a painful cramp, resulting from the muscle contracting (dystonia). This often affects the hands and feet, and can cause the feet to turn inwards. Early morning dystonia is usually caused by medication wearing off late at night or early in the morning.

Increased urination

This type of sleep disruption is called nocturia. If the urge to urinate while asleep is accompanied by an 'off' period and immobility, then getting to the toilet in time may be difficult.

Rapid eye movement (REM) sleep

Sleep is divided into REM and non-REM sleep. Normally we are partially paralysed during REM or dream sleep, so we do not act out our dreams. In Parkinson's disease (and other similar disorders) this paralysis is lost, and patients begin acting out their dreams by crying, shouting and even risk falling out of bed. Acting out violent dreams can result in their partner being hurt. This REM sleep behavioural disorder may begin many years before the first clear symptoms of Parkinson's disease, and is occasionally confused as a schizophrenic-type disorder. Fortunately, it is often easily treated.

Restless Legs Syndrome
People with Parkinson's often experience an irresistible desire to move their legs during the night, which can wake them up. This tends to be a major problem in a minority of people and dopamine drugs can offer relief. Patients may also experience pins and needles in their calf muscles.

Panic attacks and depression
People may feel panicky, which may cause rapid breathing and palpitations. This can be caused by 'off' periods or anxiety. Panic attacks may be caused by vivid dreams or hallucinations. It's important to report these problems to a neurologist who may address the issue by prescribing a drug to help. Depression and cognitive problems, such as dementia, may also cause sleep problems.

Medications
Several anti-Parkinson's drugs may also disrupt sleep. Drugs such as Symmetrel (amantadine) or Eldepryl (selegiline) can keep people awake at night. In some advanced cases, high doses of levodopa or dopamine agonist drugs can also cause insomnia. Other substances that can cause sleepless nights include caffeine, diuretics, clonidine, which is used to relieve sweating, and ephedrine, which is a stimulant drug used for postural hypotension (a drop in blood pressure when standing up, causing the person to feel light-headed and dizzy; in severe cases it can cause falls or blackouts).

Strategies for managing sleep problems

Margarita Makoutonina says there are various ways of combating insomnia: 'We try to help patients take control by using stress management and relaxation techniques.'

It's important to work out the underlying cause of sleeping problems so they can be addressed. For example, if the problem is caused by worsening symptoms, such as stiffness, pain and tremor, then the treating doctor may recommend using a longer acting anti-Parkinson's drug at bedtime. These drugs include controlled-release preparations of Sinemet and Madopar (levodopa), or the longest acting dopamine agonist, Cabaser (cabergoline) and Sifrol (pramiprexol)—although neurologists have stopped prescribing Cabaser due to cardiac valve problems and mainly use Sifrol.

If insomnia is a result of frequent urges to urinate at night, then a useful strategy is to reduce the amount of fluid intake in the evening or late afternoon, and avoid drinks such as coffee, tea or beer before bedtime. Ms Makoutonina says 'people with Parkinson's usually have difficulty moving around in bed so if they take a lot of fluid at night, they will need to go to the toilet more often. They are usually slow in getting out of bed so it becomes a vicious cycle.'

It's important to discuss sleeping problems with your GP, neurologist or allied health professional so measures can be put in place to reduce their effect.

6. RELATIONSHIPS

Being diagnosed with a chronic illness can put a strain on relationships.

For people with Parkinson's disease, the strain is likely to be greatest when someone is diagnosed in their 40s or 50s. There are difficulties in maintaining a normal healthy sex life, because erectile problems and arousal issues usually surface. People with Parkinson's disease may also feel uncomfortable with the way their body is affected. Both partners find their relationship takes on a whole new dimension.

Clinical psychologist Chris Basten says that, while some couples struggle, a diagnosis can bring other couples closer together. It gives them something to rally around and partners begin to value what they've got.

When it's a reasonably healthy relationship, a diagnosis can make the partnership stronger. When it's already fragile and marked by conflict, then the cracks open up even more.
—Dr Chris Basten

Counsellor Deb England couldn't agree more. She knows of relationships that have ended because of Parkinson's disease, but a diagnosis can also be the catalyst for separating if there are existing issues. She believes a person with Parkinson's disease needs to take some responsibility to ensure relationships with their loved ones aren't damaged. She says the patient shouldn't try to shut people out. Being totally absorbed in their illness and feeling angry about losing their 'abilities' doesn't help either. Ms England says she structures most of her counselling sessions around 'qualities' rather than 'abilities'. It's important to maintain relationships by working on the qualities that are needed to be the best partner, mum, sister or friend because these are the things that count in the long run.

> *Parkinson's disease need not impact on relationships unless you let it. There are things you can control.*
>
> —Deb England

Paula Argy, aged 39, knows all about the value of relationships, and strives to be the best mother to her two daughters. She believes her diagnosis was the catalyst for her marriage breakdown five years ago. Her children, parents and friends have helped her through the tough times. 'I feel like I get a lot of encouragement and praise from women around me'. Paula is over the trauma of the break-up and is open to dating, but has yet to meet the right person. 'It'll take a very special person to take me on,' she says.

There are also stories about patients dating people who have no knowledge of the disease, or show little interest in what it means. One woman with Parkinson's disease was asked whether she could still have sex. Another went on a date and was asked whether the disease was contagious.

Nerissa Mapes, aged 33, is single and says starting relationships can be difficult, but she's upfront about her illness very early on. She doesn't know whether that sabotages her chances, but she does think having the disease is a lot to handle in a relationship. She remembers asking one date whether he thought it was a problem. He told her it wasn't, so long as she didn't bore him with the details. While Nerissa

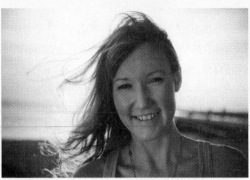

Nerissa Mapes

does worry about the future, she says she won't let her fears take over. She has a wonderful group of friends and remains positive.

> *I prefer people to ask me questions about the illness.*
> *Some people are really shocked when they find out I have*
> *Parkinson's disease, as I'm really young and they might feel*
> *sorry for me and get sad. When people think of Parkinson's,*
> *they have this picture of an old man with the shakes. But*
> *here I am, a young woman wearing stilettos.*
>
> —Nerissa Mapes

Peter McWilliam, 67, admits Parkinson's disease is not a fun disease to be around, but he doesn't blame his condition for the breakdown of his marriage seven years ago. 'My wife lives nearby and she's very supportive', he says.

Pauline England cares for her husband Brian, who was diagnosed 20 years ago. They've been married for more than five decades.

> *The most important thing is to learn to laugh at it. That's*
> *what we've done. With all our problems over the years,*
> *people sometimes think we're nuts I'm sure. We look at each*

other and see something funny and we laugh together. I think
that's an important thing. If you can learn to laugh at the
flipping disease it's a big thing.

Have a good laugh and don't get too bogged down in the
disease. You've got it ... so make the best of it.

—Pauline England, 73, wife and carer of Parkinson's patient

Carer Sue Rance agrees humour is a good way of dealing
with the many challenges that come with the illness. She's been
married to Phil for many years, and when her husband experienced major behavioural problems because of his Parkinson's
medication, they nearly got divorced. Now their relationship
is back on track and she sees the funny side of awkward situations. 'When he's completely off and he can't get undressed,
we'll make a joke of it.'

It's a lot easier if you become informed. If I hadn't pushed
to get information about the agonist medications or kept my
association with Parkinson's NSW, I don't know where we'd
be right now. Phil was pretty keen to get divorced. His family
is in the UK and he was talking seriously of going back there.
If he'd continued taking the agonist medication, I don't know
where we'd be right now. I certainly feel that knowledge is
very important.

—Sue Rance, wife and carer

Another carer, Dan Mongan, says he and his wife Fay have
remained positive, despite the adversities. Fay, 75, took a turn
for the worse recently, when she could no longer do her favourite things, like cook and sew. But new medication changed that.
The couple have two children, five grandchildren and a strong
network of friends. Fay remains close to her sister and another
friend, both bridesmaids at her 1955 wedding. 'Fay's sister lives
nearby,' says Dan. 'She comes over up to three times a week. The

other bridesmaid lives in Wollongong and never misses sending us cards, and we're having lunch tomorrow. There's another friend who drives us to hospital every time we have to go.'

Dan's advice to people who are newly diagnosed is to be positive in your outlook on life. 'You've still got life ahead of you so plan every day living it and enjoying it. We used to like going to the pictures. We had a trip to Disneyland and Hong Kong. We've had a good life and so have the kids. There is something to live for no matter how bad your circumstances are.'

> *There's an old saying: I used to complain about having no shoes until I met a man who had no feet. There's so much truth to that. There's always someone who is worse off.*
> —Dan Mongan, husband and carer

Sue Rance's Story

Phil was diagnosed with Parkinson's disease in 1997 at the age of 46. The year before his diagnosis, Phil suffered from an anxiety disorder which we were told later is often the beginnings of Parkinson's disease. Though this improved, he began to feel particularly tired and was dragging his left leg.

As soon as he was diagnosed with Parkinson's disease, he was put on the dopamine agonist Permax. I believe the start of this drug is what led to major personality changes in Phil, which was not only devastating but nearly led to the breakdown of our marriage. Phil began to gamble a lot and was always betting on the pokies. Fortunately, I controlled the finances so he never had access to large amounts of money. He also became hypersexual and started borrowing blue movies. There was also an aggressive streak I had never seen before. He became extremely religious to the point he decided to be baptised and confirmed. His actions were completely out of character.

In 2001 Phil was diagnosed with bipolar disorder. I sought

comfort in counselling and found it incredibly helpful. It saved me from going 'berserk'. I also spoke to a woman who'd been on Permax who suffered manic episodes of depression. She told me when she came off the drug, things returned to normal.

I decided to approach Phil's psychiatrist and neurologist about taking him off the medication. Eventually, after seven years on Permax, he was taken off the drug. Immediately I saw an improvement. He was far less aggressive, far less hypersexual and far less interested in gambling. You wouldn't know he was the same person.

When Phil was diagnosed in 1997 we became extremely close. We always had a good relationship, but his Parkinson's made us closer. We were committed to working as a team. But that all changed when he went on the medication.

We have worked really hard dealing with Parkinson's and its problems to get where we are today. We have no kids and our family is based in the UK, so we had to find our own support in Australia. I found counselling unbelievably helpful and am adamant I wouldn't have got through the problems without it. I have many good girlfriends to talk to and my sister in the UK always provides a listening ear. In 2005 Phil became more accepting of his diagnosis but it was a long journey to get there.

Nowadays I work once a week as a volunteer for Parkinson's NSW. I believe people are better off making contact with support groups. Phil belongs to the Young Men's Support group and, although he doesn't say much, he usually gets something out of being there with others who are experiencing the same disease in different ways. The partners meet at the same time for a friendly chat and to give each other support. I believe these things really help when keeping relationships together.

Sexual dysfunction

Sexual dysfunction is common among patients with neurological disorders, including Parkinson's disease.[1] Studies suggest that the problem is one of the most demoralising and disabling features of the disease.

Erectile dysfunction is one of the most commonly reported problems for males (see Table 6.1). It can happen because of the effects of nerve signals from the brain or poor blood circulation. Men also report sexual dissatisfaction, premature ejaculation and difficulties reaching orgasm as common problems.

Table 6.1 Sexual problems in men who have Parkinson's disease[2]

Type of sexual problem	Participants affected/Number in study	Percentage affected
Erectile dysfunction	26/38	68.4
Dissatisfaction with sex life	28/43	65.1
Premature ejaculation	13/32	40.6
Trouble reaching orgasm	15/38	39.5
Difficulties ejaculating	9/33	27.3
Sexual desire (seldom/ never)	10/43	23.3
Stopped having sex	10/43	23.3

Note: The average age of subjects was 63 years; mean duration of Parkinson's disease symptoms was 8.9 years. Most subjects were taking levodopa or dopamine agonists or both. Source: Bonner & Royter. (2004) *Journal of Sex & Marital Therapy*. 30: pp 95–105. Reproduced with permission

When rating their level of sexual dysfunction, women put difficulties with arousal at the top of their list, followed by problems with reaching orgasm, then reduced sexual desire (or libido).

Table 6.2 Sexual problems in women who have Parkinson's disease[3]

Type of sexual problem	Participants affected/Number in study	Percentage affected
Difficulties getting aroused	21/24	87.5
Trouble reaching orgasm	18/24	75.0
Sexual desire (seldom/never)	15/32	46.9
Dissatisfaction with sex life	12/32	37.5
Stopped having sex	7/32	21.9
Painful sex	3/24	12.5

Source: Bonner & Royter. (2004) *Journal of Sex & Marital Therapy*. 30: pp 95–105. Reproduced with permission

These factors can greatly impact on the level of sexual activity and can add stress to relationships. Other health conditions, the use of medications and advanced stages of Parkinson's disease can all make the problem worse. Hypersexuality from levodopa and dopamine agonists can also occur.

In the past, neurologists haven't paid much attention to intimacy issues, and patients have been reluctant to share information about their love life.[4]

Strategies for managing sexual dysfunction

Occupational therapist Margarita Makoutonina says neurologists often don't have time to deal with the subject and some patients aren't even aware that their sexual problems might stem from their medical condition or treatment. They might also be embarrassed so they're unlikely to raise it with their specialist. 'People need to explore the changes [in their lives after diagnosis] and discuss their feelings with their partner. One man with Parkinson's disease thought his wife wasn't interested in him any more, when in fact she was going through menopause. I do try to remind couples that stress, anxiety and depression also affect intimacy.' Anti-depressants may reduce sex drive so advice should be sought to help tackle both problems.

'I talk to a patient about the easiest position for sexual intercourse, and other ways of maintaining intimacy to help their relationship,' Margarita says.

Treatments for impotence, such as Viagra, might be needed in some cases. Viagra has been shown to be safe and effective in men with Parkinson's disease.

Supporting the carer

When Muhammad Ali and I married, he had already been diagnosed with Parkinson's syndrome. Later that diagnosis was changed to Parkinson's disease, which meant Muhammad's condition would progress as time went on. Never having met anyone with PD, I felt alone. There was no one for me to talk to who was in a similar situation. Looking back, I wish I'd had a better understanding of the disease as well as the role of the caregiver. I have since learned a lot about care giving that, had I known years ago, would have made life easier for me and my husband.

—Lonnie Ali[5]

Carers can go through exactly the same emotions as their loved one when a diagnosis is made. There can be a mixture of shock, anger and resentment. What happens to life plans? What happens to retirement plans? Will I have to quit work if the symptoms get worse? What about our financial future?

While struggling with their own feelings, there's no denying how important the caregiver's role will be in the years ahead as the disease progresses. Carers are vital in ensuring a patient can properly manage in the home and maintain independence. Without that support, the challenges of the disease will be more difficult to overcome.

Paula Argy, aged 39, is worried about who will be left to care for her in the event she's no longer able to cope at home. 'My parents are getting older. They're in their mid 60s. My husband isn't around and I worry about my children. One of my biggest fears is my children [having to look] after me. I'm not opposed to going into a nursing home. I'd rather that than burden my family. Though I'm aware there is not a lot of choice for younger people in care facilities.'

Sue Rance describes her initial reaction when her husband Phil was diagnosed 12 years ago at the age of 46: 'We were in shock, complete shock and denial. This definitely can't be happening to us. It just came out of the blue like something had hit us.'

She says Phil gradually got worse, and was forced to give up work as a painter and decorator because his balance was badly affected. If he had a desk job with less stress maybe he could have continued working for longer. 'Driving became too much for him so he doesn't drive at all now, so I've taken over.

I've always taken care of finances so that hasn't changed. But gradually I've had to do more.'

Sue said she gave up work in 2005, which made life easier all round. 'I drive Phil to his appointments and activities. I do all the shopping and all of the cooking.'

An occupational therapist visited their home to provide advice on any changes that would make their life more comfortable. She recommended having a bedside commode, so Phil could avoid having to walk to the toilet in the middle of the night. But there weren't too many adjustments that were required.

Sue says that Phil remains relatively independent and he prefers to do things himself. He tries very hard to have a shower when he's 'on'. He can do that without too much trouble. When he's 'off', he can't shower at all. Sue says if his symptoms deteriorate, other help might be needed. 'Parkinson's is so individual, one day can be totally different to the next. The worst-case scenario is I may have to dress Phil or help him in the middle of the night to get out of bed to use the commode,' she says.

> *One of the best pieces of advice I got from my counsellor was don't be a martyr, it doesn't work. I often think of that.*
>
> —Sue Rance

Occupational therapist Margarita Makoutonina says carers play a vital role in assisting their loved one. 'It's not only the patient who is diagnosed with Parkinson's disease, the whole family is involved.' Margarita says that the more the family is involved from day one and the more they learn, the better their quality of life will be.

To do a good job, the carer needs to have a lot of understanding of the challenges that come with the disease. Carers also need to:[6]

- learn when to help and when not to
- allow time for the person to do things on their own, without hurrying
- learn not to take over (don't speak for them)
- find out where to go for help for tips on daily living
- adopt survival strategies
- be honest in the relationship.

As the disease progresses, there's no denying that the carer's responsibilities become harder, which can lead to frustration, depression and sleeping problems. If the carer feels fatigued, they need to get help to ensure their health is not compromised. Signs of fatigue include:

- a tendency to continually ignore or postpone taking care of their own health needs
- feeling isolated ('Nobody knows or understands what is really going on with us')
- feeling anxious and uncertain about the future, which can trigger verbal or even physical abuse of the patient
- feeling angry at the person or situation, which is often followed by feelings of guilt
- tiredness or feelings of exhaustion not relieved by sleep
- emotional strain or stress, which often leads to physical symptoms developing
- an inability to concentrate or make decisions
- bitterness toward friends or relatives who 'should help more'
- the use of alcohol or drugs to alleviate stress
- depression, despair or feelings of hopelessness.

What the carers say

Sue Rance says she was advised early on to look after herself. 'I do work on that. I go to counselling, do Pilates, and see an osteopath for knee and back problems.' Sue has a subscription to go to eight concerts a year, which gives her a break and she likes to catch up with women friends for coffee.

> *Phil would like me with him 24 hours a day, but he totally understands that wouldn't be good for him and it wouldn't be good for me. I know if I'm more relaxed, I can be so much nicer with him, rather than feel tired, fed up and cranky. I find that I cope a lot better if I look after myself.*
>
> —Sue Rance

Carer Pauline England, aged 73, says coping with the finances was hard to deal with initially. Her husband Brian was diagnosed 20 years ago, and she has gradually learned to take over the tasks he used to be in charge of. 'I always say we've had a complete role reversal. He was the boss, and now I make all the decisions, which was extremely hard to start with. I had to learn to do all the banking and paying of bills. They were all of his jobs. It was difficult for him to let go and it was hard for me to take them from him.'

> *The impact [on the carer] can be enormous and there is a lot of role reversal that muddies the water. Especially if the man has to suddenly organise the household, or the woman suddenly becomes the breadwinner.*
>
> —Deb England, counsellor

Brian England handed over his car keys to Pauline ten years ago after they were nearly involved in a collision. Pauline says: 'All the things he's had to let go has been difficult for him and it has been difficult for me to watch.'

Brian's health has deteriorated in the past two years, since he contracted an infection while in hospital. His wife Pauline used to supervise him in the home before he became sick.

'You don't want to take all their independence away from them. I would be there when it was shower time. If he needed help then he'd ask for it.' But nowadays she uses a group called St Ives, whose carers come into the home to help Brian shower and dress everyday. Pauline says she might have managed on her own but it would have been exhausting.

When Brian ventures out once a week with a group it gives Pauline the chance to do the shopping and other chores. The bus picks him up every Wednesday, so this is the day she has to herself.

For emotional support, Pauline relies on two women friends and one of her four sons, who lives nearby and is also good at providing help.

Dan Mongan, aged 77, has been married to Fay for more than 50 years. She was formally diagnosed with Parkinson's in the mid 1990s, but her symptoms started to emerge a decade before. Recently she was put onto a new treatment Apomine, which requires daily infusions.

> I had the community nurses come over to show me how to put the needle in each morning. I never thought I'd be able to put a needle into somebody else, particularly my wife. I used to go and get a blood test and just shrink.
>
> This is something I have to do, I'm obliged to do, and I owe her to do. When she wakes up at two, three or four in the morning I have to take her to the toilet. To me, ten years ago, it would have been something demeaning. Now it's something I have to do to help her. It's the same with showering.

Dan says he has become a different person, taking charge of domestic tasks such as shopping. He was an accountant by trade and worked for the TAB for 28 years. At age 65, he was given the opportunity to work part-time at a legal firm to deliver mail. The woman asked whether he was up to pushing a trolley. He said, 'I go to the supermarket and push a trolley, and have to pay. You're going to pay me to push a trolley now.' Dan had to give up that job six years ago after Fay's condition deteriorated and the demands at home became more of a priority.

The cost of medical supplies concern him, given he receives a small carer's allowance of $105 a fortnight. Recently carers were given a financial boost of only $1.03 extra a fortnight with their allowance. Dan was also unhappy with having to spend a lot of time on the road to pick up Fay's Apomine medication from the hospital pharmacy. Instead of being able to obtain her medication at a hospital close to their home in Sydney's southwest, he had to drive to a hospital near the city, and then wait 45 minutes while staff prepared the drug. After complaining to the NSW health minister, the system was changed and Dan was allowed to access her treatment from a hospital closer to home. What used to be a three-hour round trip for Dan, has now been reduced to 50 minutes.

Dan and Fay were also paying about $780 a year for needles, patches and alcohol wipes. They didn't know until recently that district nurses provided these consumables for free. Their power bill is about $1800 a year, so everything starts to add up. They get a state pensioner's rebate on their power bill ($130 a year) but they still have to pay 10 per cent GST. Dan has written to the federal government, suggesting carers not be charged GST on their electricity bills. In NSW, people with Multiple Sclerosis or Parkinson's get a state rebate on their power bill amounting to $32.50 every quarter.

While Dan's happy with the level of support he receives from friends and family, he says accessing medical supplies and the extra costs that come with a chronic illness do not make life any easier. He believes that both state and federal governments can do more to help alleviate the financial burden, and make the medical system more efficient.

But he puts things in perspective. 'I get the pension and my outlook on life is this: I get half a bed and two home-cooked meals a day so I'm doing fine. I'm a 77-year-old with arthritis but I've got friends, family, a good wife and good grandchildren. What more could you want?'

An expert's view

Occupational therapist Dr Anne Hillman interviewed 25 people who have Parkinson's disease and their partners. She found that many of the husbands and wives didn't see themselves as carers. 'A lot of them rejected that label. They would say things like, "Of course I'm going to look after him/her, it's part of my role as the partner. It's fine, it's not a problem".'

It was only in the later stages that partners saw themselves as having two roles: one as the partner, the other as a carer. It was often the cognitive changes that develop late in the disease that prompted partners to accept their dual role. Dr Hillman says: 'In particular, that related to dementia. Partners were saying things like "I still love her/him very much, but I've lost that relationship we once had." So it wasn't the physical disability that brought about change.'

Advice for carers

Counsellor Deb England says the welfare of carers worries her enormously. When they can get out and obtain some respite, there isn't much of a problem. But community respite is hard to come by. And a lot of guilt buttons are pushed when they decide to take a break. Deb says 'it's not an act of selfishness. You're the linchpin. You have to accept whatever help is available so you don't become ill.'

> *Taking care of yourself isn't an act of selfishness. It's an act of keeping all the balls in the air.*
>
> —Deb England

Carers need encouragement and recognition, so they feel validated. They also need:[7]

- information
- a listening ear
- support so they can express their frustrations
- easy access to treatment for themselves
- good communication with health professionals
- quality time away
- access to respite care
- a good night's sleep (this is very rare and is a big issue for carers)
- to look after themselves and their health
- a sense of humour
- pampering from time to time.

Professor Robert Iansek says that the role of the carer is extremely important in helping people with Parkinson's achieve a more normal life. 'We need to focus on the carers, train them, support them, and look at ways of keeping people at home as long as possible,' he says.

Carers may be at increased risk of depression so it's important they eat well, exercise and get enough sleep. They should also allocate time during the day to relax and do something enjoyable.

Dan Mongan shares this advice with fellow carers: 'Keep positive and if there's help, accept it. It's important to your health that you reach out.'

A lady was very badly affected by Parkinson's disease and her husband cared for her. He was diagnosed with an aggressive form of cancer. One day he had returned home from shopping and was berated by his wife for getting the wrong hand cream. The family's thinking, for goodness

sake, Dad is going to be dead in a minute and here you are
banging on about hand cream.

—Deb England

Useful addresses
Carers Australia
  www.carersaustralia.com.au
  1800 242 636

Commonwealth Respite & Carelink Centres
  www.commcarelink.health.gov.au
  1800 052 222

Government Assistance enquiries (disability, sickness, carers)
  www.centrelink.gov.au
  13 27 17

7. THE FUTURE

Parkinson's is not really a uniform disease. In fact it's probably many diseases so we'll be lucky to find one treatment that fits all, like the present drug therapy which improves some of the symptoms.

—Professor Garth Nicholson, neurogeneticist

Millions of dollars is being spent around the world to try to find a cure for Parkinson's disease, or at least enhance current treatments to improve quality of life. Scientists are working on providing better drugs, especially for patients who have limited options in the advanced stages of the disease.

Deep brain stimulation is proving to be one of the biggest advances in the last decade. The invasive surgical procedure is not for everyone but improvements in technology will see this technique be more widely used in the future.

Much has been said in the popular media about the potential benefits of stem cell therapy, and researchers continue to investigate this avenue along with gene therapy as future treatment options.

Better drug therapies

I heard there were 26 new drugs being tested for Parkinson's disease. I think drug therapies are going to become more sophisticated as our understanding of the disease becomes deeper.

—Dr Bryce Vissel, scientist

Levodopa has been the mainstay treatment for people with Parkinson's for nearly half a century. It can dramatically improve many of the debilitating symptoms, while allowing people to get on with their lives. However, the treatment usually loses its effect after years of someone taking the drug. It becomes less reliable and can have side effects, such as uncontrolled involuntary movements.

Other drugs have been developed as an alternative or to be used in combination with levodopa. Some of the new treatments include Neupro, a dopamine agonist drug, which is the only skin patch that's available in Australia to treat symptoms of Parkinson's disease. The patch allows the drug to be slowly absorbed through the bloodstream over 24 hours. This treatment is not currently subsidised under the Pharmaceutical Benefits Scheme but may be in the future.

Another development is the drug Duodopa. Provided in a gel form, it is administered continuously by a pump directly into the small intestine to allow more rapid absorption. This leads to a more continuous flow of medication to the brain. The drug contains levodopa and carbidopa (as found in Sinemet): the latter helps ensure the largest amount of levodopa reaches the brain. The treatment minimises involuntary body movements by keeping the levodopa concentration relatively constant. This means motor function can be kept at a stable level and at best, avoid 'off' periods.[1] This treatment is not currently subsidised under the Pharmaceutical Benefits Scheme. It's considered a good means of delivering the L-dopa and carbidopa combination, but it is very expensive.

Apomorphine is another advance for people who have exhausted mainstay treatment and is available on the PBS through hospital pharmacies only. Dr Jeremy Playfer from the Parkinson's Disease Society (UK), says:

> *Because it can be injected, [apomorphine] works more quickly than tablets. This rapid effect means that people have better control over debilitating symptoms for much longer. Apomorphine can be given as intermittent injections or via an infusion under the skin. This constant infusion helps to overcome the fluctuations associated with levodopa. To date, apomorphine has helped many thousands of people manage their disabling symptoms and regain their independence.*[2]

The use of items such as patches, syringes and pumps to deliver medication is not subsidised by the Australian government. This means highly effective new treatments are limited to those who can afford them. In May 2009 Parkinson's Australia made a submission to the Department of Health and Ageing, calling for a scheme that provides access to essential products and continuous infusion devices to deliver Parkinson's medication (along similar lines as the Diabetes Services Scheme, which provides a range of products such as free insulin syringes, pen needles and subsidised insulin pumps). The group also urged the government to increase access to new treatment options, such as deep brain stimulation, which is too expensive for many. Even with private health insurance, patients are generally left $15,000 to $20,000 out of pocket. 'We believe this inequity in access to treatment to be discriminatory and unacceptable. Parkinson's is an illness where timely access to new pharmaceuticals and new treatment options is crucial to the wellbeing of the sufferer.'[3]

Bill's story

Bill has been living with Parkinson's for 27 years.

Levodopa worked really well for me for about 20 years. But all that changed a few years ago. My tremor became worse and my whole body would shake uncontrollably. I was finding it more and more difficult to do simple tasks such as buttoning my shirt or tying my shoelaces. Walking was a struggle. Without warning, my feet would feel glued to the ground. I would be helpless and unable to take another step for minutes. My specialist said that the levodopa tablets were no longer controlling my symptoms so he put me on apomorphine as well. I now have a special pump on a belt around my waist, which slowly releases apomorphine into my body 24 hours a day. I have my life back again and can do things I enjoy, like playing chess and gardening.

— 'Four Decades of Discovery', Parkinson's Disease Society, UK

Refining current treatments

I'm more excited about deep brain stimulation and refining the process than stem cell research.

—Dr Chris Basten, clinical psychologist

I think we're going to see more developments and better results with deep brain stimulation.

—Dr Richard Bittar, neurosurgeon

Deep brain stimulation (DBS) is considered the biggest development in treating people with Parkinson's disease in recent times. Many people have been treated using electrical stimulation and had remarkable results. DBS can help reduce a patient's debilitating symptoms, so they can regain their quality of life. Dozens of trials are being carried out around the world to further investigate its effectiveness and to improve the technique.

Melbourne neurosurgeon Dr Richard Bittar says we're going to see big improvements in DBS technology:

We're starting to see rechargeable batteries come in so patients
don't need to change their batteries every three to four years.
We're going to see different types of electrodes. The wires we
put in the brain are going to be much more sophisticated in
terms of the way they allow us to direct the current. We will
see patients have a better chance of a good outcome.

Dr Bittar says a better understanding of the way the brain functions will also help in choosing new targets. He says targets for
deep brain stimulation further in the brain tend to be important in patients who have problems with balance and walking.
Researchers have done studies in monkeys and the procedure
will be tested in some humans who have Parkinson's and have
balance problems that are difficult to treat. He says better electrodes are being developed, and in the future they will be placed
in more positions, depending on the patient's needs.

In Perth, neurosurgeon Christopher Lind has adopted a
technique that avoids the need for patients to remain awake
during the procedure. Surgeons use implantable plastic guide
tubes and perform MRI brain scans during the operation under
general anaesthesia. This technique, developed by Professor
Steven Gill of the Frenchay Hospital in Bristol, in Britain, helps
ensure accuracy in placing the electrodes. Professor Lind says
his team has successfully used this method for implanting electrodes for DBS in the treatment of Parkinson's disease. For the
patients treated, the DBS electrode was delivered to within 1.5
millimetres of the planned target in the brain.[4]

I think there are going to be many potential areas of
improvement in the way we treat these patients.

—Dr Richard Bittar

Dr Bittar says one of the main benefits for patients of deep
brain stimulation is that the procedure is reversible, unlike the

cruder techniques of the past, where doctors literally burned a hole in the brain. In addition, the treatment is adjustable and non-destructive. That means patients are eligible for new therapies if they become available in five to ten years time.

Improving diagnosis

Sydney neurologist Dr Victor Fung says it's thought the disease starts to develop at least several years before the symptoms emerge. About 50 to 70 per cent of dopamine neurons have been lost before symptoms first show. So someone who starts to show symptoms has only 30 per cent of their dopamine neurons left. He says we need a therapy that prevents the death of the surviving dopamine neurons: 'But even before a therapy can be used, a person needs to be diagnosed properly. That's why it's important to come up with a test that's economical for patients.' There are currently no diagnostic tests available in Australia.

American researchers have developed a method to track the progression of Parkinson's in patients who are in the early stages of the disease. It uses positron emission tomography (PET) imaging techniques. These techniques allow the researchers to examine dopamine transporter binding, a measure of dopamine levels in the brains of people with Parkinson's disease and in healthy individuals. They have found that the start of movement problems in people who have Parkinson's disease is accompanied by a 70 per cent loss of dopamine in the brain. PET imaging of Parkinson's patients shows hyperactivity in some brain regions prior to treatment, probably resulting from the loss of dopamine, which normally acts to quieten down these areas. Deep brain stimulation reduces this hyperactivity.[5]

Other researchers are using single photon emission computed tomography (SPECT) and magnetic resonance imaging (MRI) to examine the brain's nicotine receptors which respond to the neurotransmitter acetylcholine. Previous studies have shown changes in the acetylcholine system in PD patients. These changes tend to be more pronounced in patients with dementia. The current study should clarify how acetylcholine interacts with other neurotransmitters in people with PD, and may lead to new ways of diagnosing or treating the disease.

Dr Fung says the use of fluoro-levodopa scans and SPECT, which confirm reduced dopamine in the basal ganglia, are available in Europe and the United States but not in Australia. 'They're too expensive to be used as a screening tool and are mainly used for the purpose of research,' he says. 'However, they can be very helpful in diagnosis when a neurologist is not sure whether someone has Parkinson's disease.'

Smell tests

> *I have to be careful with cooking. Quite often I'll leave the hot plate on and when I'm on the phone I forget that I was cooking. You lose your sense of smell.*
>
> —Karen Rowland, diagnosed in her 40s

Loss of smell is one of the more common symptoms that can develop early in people with Parkinson's disease. Knowing this, scientists are developing ways of identifying people who are experiencing these problems and may be at risk of having the disease.

In 2003 Sydney researchers identified the type of odours patients have difficulty picking up. Of the 12 odours tested, they found that gasoline, banana, pineapple, smoke and cinnamon were the ones that patients had trouble with. The authors suggested that the specific problems they recognised could be used in the development of smell tests designed to help in the early diagnosis of Parkinson's disease—perhaps even before any symptoms appeared.[6]

In 2006, another Australian team adopted a 'scratch and smell' test to identify people at risk of developing brain disorders before the appearance of any symptoms.

University of Melbourne researchers discovered a link between the inability to detect and identify smells, and a range of brain disorders, including Alzheimer's, Huntington's and Parkinson's disease, schizophrenia and obsessive–compulsive disorder. People who took part in the smell tests were asked to identify odours such as coffee, roses, oranges and petrol. Those who later went on to develop a brain disorder or mental illness had trouble correctly answering more than half the questions asked of them.

Professor Christos Pantelis, from the University of Melbourne, told Channel Nine that a test of this kind would provide doctors with extra information to help diagnose a patient. He said smell ability provided unique information about brain structure and function. 'Mental illness can arrest the full maturation (development) of the frontal lobe, while degenerative illness can damage it. This area of the brain is used to analyse and identify smells so an abnormal sense of smell may indicate problems in the "thinking" area of the brain,' he said.

Researching the genetics of Parkinson's

Scientists around the world have spent decades trying to unravel the mysteries of Parkinson's disease and understand why people stop producing enough dopamine in the brain.

The discovery of new genes linked to the disease is helping provide important clues. Everyone once believed Parkinson's disease was entirely caused by environmental factors, but it's now known that a combination of genes can increase risk.

Two recent discoveries have shown that mutations in the PINK gene lead to a rare form of inherited Parkinson's, and another defect gene, called LRRK2, has also been linked to the disease.

'These genes appear to be important for everyone and keep the nerve cells working smoothly. By understanding how defects in the genes damage nerve cells, we can help all people with Parkinson's,' says Professor Nick Wood, consultant neurologist.[7]

He says the next phase of research will involve looking at how these genes operate normally compared with when they're defective.

Two mutated genes known to cause inherited forms of Parkinson's disease are also associated with the more common, sporadic forms where there is no family history of the disease. Scientists in the US showed that mutations in the SNCA and MAPT genes, both present in the general population, are risk factors for non-inherited Parkinson's disease.

Evidence is also mounting that environmental factors are important in determining whether someone who is carrying a genetic mutation will end up with Parkinson's disease. 'For most people, it's going to be the sum of a number of different factors—both genetic predisposition and environmental exposures—that will determine whether or not a certain individual develops Parkinson's disease,' says American neurologist Dr Caroline Tanner.[8]

Sydney scientist Dr Bryce Vissel says the genes that have been identified will give scientists a better handle on what causes the disease, because it will allow scientists 'to start engineering genes in mice, and see what happens so that we begin to understand what mechanisms contribute to cell loss. There's a general thought that there's a common pathway that goes wrong. If we're lucky to find all the mutant genes, we could find a common pathway,' he says.

> *As we get to understand the genetics better we might start to understand that there are various forms that might lead to specific therapies based on the genetic strain.*
>
> —Dr Bryce Vissel

Australian researchers are developing an affordable blood test to identify people with genetic mutations. At the moment, genetic testing is mostly used for research, but that could soon change as scientists work on producing a test that's more affordable to patients. Sydney neurogeneticist Garth Nicholson says his team is developing a blood test that can identify '80 per cent of the known Parkinson's gene mutations'. He says:

> *Hopefully it would cost less than a few thousand dollars. As far as I know, no one in the world has succeeded in doing this but we're trying.*
>
> *People might want to know about this information because in the future, a preventative or treatment might come up for families with the known genetic defect. They might also want to use IVF to ensure they don't pass on the gene.*

However, he adds, the diagnostic test won't give a full picture of the affected genes because there are a number of genetic mutations that are still unknown.

> *I'm very optimistic that treatments will come up probably in the not too distant future. They may only apply to certain sub-groups of Parkinson's disease. You'd be very lucky to get one that works for the whole lot.*
>
> —Professor Garth Nicholson

Researchers in Melbourne have created a genetic test for Parkinson's disease using a tiny silicon chip. It involves extracting DNA from a saliva sample, then putting those gene sequences onto the chip to identify any mutations relating to Parkinson's disease.

The test was developed in 2007, after 530 people who had Parkinson's took part in the study to test the accuracy of the device. A scientist at the Florey Neuroscience Institutes said the test would cost about $500, which is relatively inexpensive.

Dr Qiao-Xin Li and his team from the University of Melbourne, along with Professor Malcolm Horne from the Florey Neuroscience Institutes, found that people who had Parkinson's disease had altered levels of alpha-synuclein protein in their blood. The protein is a product of the SNCA gene. The Institutes have also developed another test, using blood samples, to measure this protein, which is released from the brain. Professor Horne says, 'About a third of people with Parkinson's disease have abnormal levels of the protein.' He compares this discovery with the development of glucose testing for diabetes.

'One of the big breakthroughs was the discovery that abnormal glucose is related to diabetes. So if you say, here's a protein that is always up or altered in Parkinson's disease, then you can pour your efforts into working out why that protein is messed up.'

Researchers often need the help of people with Parkinson's disease to carry out their work. Some states have a register that collects information from patients, so their DNA and blood samples can be analysed. Many volunteers are also willing to take part in other studies to investigate issues such as pain, behavioural problems and the welfare of carers.

Professor Nicholson says, 'I'm interested in finding families with Parkinson's disease to look at new genes involved in the disease. Every one of them will help us screen for drugs that will target different people affected by Parkinson's.'

Professor Andrew Singleton, of the National Institutes of Health, says:

> *With this better understanding of the underlying genetic variants involved in the progress of this disorder, we have more insight into the causes and underlying biology of this disease. We hope this new understanding will one day provide us with strategies to delay, or even prevent, the development of Parkinson's disease.*[9]

Sergey Brin Starts Study After Finding
He Has Parkinson's Mutation

Sergey Brin, the co-founder of Google, is to spend millions of dollars on an innovative genetic study of Parkinson's disease after learning that he has a genetic mutation.

Mr Brin's mother has the disease and when he took a test last year, he learnt that he has inherited a mutation of a gene called LRRK2, which raises his risk of developing the condition to between 20 and 80 per cent.

The genetic study will invite 10,000 Parkinson's patients to have their DNA analysed for a token fee to investigate inherited and environmental factors that contribute to the disease and to advance research into new treatments.

Their genetic information will be compared to healthy customers of 23andMe, a company that charges $620 for DNA scans that assess people's chances of developing 105 diseases from breast cancer to baldness.

The donation by 35-year-old Sergey Brin, who is married to Anne Wojcicki, the co-founder of 23andMe, means that Parkinson's patients will pay just $18 for the company's service.

The goal is to identify DNA variations that are more common among people with Parkinson's than among healthy controls, which could be linked to its development.

Both Parkinson's patients and 23andMe's customers will be asked to fill in detailed lifestyle questionnaires which could reveal how environmental triggers interact with genes to cause the disease.

'We can make significant progress in understanding Parkinson's Disease if individuals join together and contribute their personal experiences to scientific research,' Mr Brin said.

'Basic discoveries can definitely lead to new treatments and we hope any information we find gets used for new therapies.'

'Secondly, if there is a genetic component to Parkinson's, nothing is more profitable to individuals than helping out their children.'

Parkinson's patients will be invited through the Parkinson's Institute and the Michael J. Fox Foundation, a research charity founded by the actor.

—Adapted from *Times Online*, 12 March 2009, Mark Henderson

Other research developments

More is being understood about the underlying biology of Parkinson's disease and how the brain deals with changes.

At the Garvan Institute of Medical Research, researchers say it's likely that inflammation aggravates existing damage in the central nervous system of people who have Parkinson's or Alzheimer's disease or motor neuron disease.

Their experiments on mice revealed that nerve cells in the brain produce an anti-inflammatory molecule that allows the brain to repair itself. Dr Bryce Vissel says, 'We found high levels of a molecule known as Activin A whenever regeneration occurred. This was especially interesting because the molecule is released from nerve cells. Through more experiments, we came to realise that the main action of Activin A was to block inflammation in the brain after degeneration or injury.'

Dr Vissel and his colleagues believe that chronic inflammation probably creates a harmful feedback loop that prevents the brain from healing: 'Clearly the brain's anti-inflammatory response is not working well in chronic neurodegenerative diseases.'

Dr Vissel adds, 'There are a number of studies showing that people who take non-steroidal anti-inflammatory drugs have a lower risk of Alzheimer's and Parkinson's disease.'

The team believes that if further research confirms their findings, Activin A and its derivatives should be investigated for their potential in Parkinson's therapy. Dr Vissel says there is already evidence that people taking ibuprofen (an anti-inflammatory) have a lower risk of Parkinson's disease.

Scientists overseas have also looked at the link between inflammation in the brain and Parkinson's. In France, scientists found that rogue immune cells entering the brain may cause Parkinson's disease. They looked for the presence in the brain tissues of a particular type of immune cell, T-cell, that is directly affected by the disease. They found that T-cells had gathered in brain samples from deceased patients, and at an earlier stage in mice bred to develop the disease. When mice lacked T-cells, the rate of nerve cell death was significantly slower. Researchers believe their findings could lead to the development of new drugs to slow the progress of the disease.[10]

Stem cells

Stem cells are unspecialised cells in the body that can divide and turn into types of cells such as skin, bone and blood. There are also different types of stem cells. These range from embryonic cells, which may be able to turn into any cell within the body, to forms of stem cells that have partially developed and may only form one type of tissue, for example blood cells. Stem cells can be sourced from the early stages of embryo formation, aborted foetuses, blood cells from the umbilical cord and even bone marrow. These cells offer hope because of their ability to replace a wide variety of damaged cells in the body, and treat conditions like heart failure, diabetes, spinal injuries and Parkinson's disease. Research and knowledge in this field has moved ahead in leaps and bounds over the last ten years. In Parkinson's it's hoped that stem cells can be grown and turned into new, healthy dopamine-producing cells, to replace the cells lost in the brain. Stem cells could also be used to develop and test new drug treatments, by growing them in the laboratory to see if the drugs are toxic or not. The use of stem cells to trial new drugs is regarded as a superior option because the cells are more likely than animal models to mimic the response of human tissue to new drugs.[11]

According to Professor Niall Quinn, consultant neurologist:

> *In the early 1990s the UK Parkinson's Disease Society helped fund early cell transplantation trials in a small group of people with Parkinson's. Human foetal nerve cells were implanted into people's brains. Although the surgery did not work for most people, two patients showed remarkable improvements. Overall the results were unpredictable and caused disabling side effects in some people. However, researchers are still learning from those initial trials, which have provided the groundwork for further research. Moving forward, the focus for future transplants will be ultimately on stem cells—an area in which the Society invests significantly.*
>
> —'Four Decades of Discovery', Parkinson's Disease Society UK

Neurogeneticist Professor Garth Nicholson believes stem cell therapy is not going to deliver a cure for patients at present. He says there are risks associated with placing growing stem cells of any sort in someone's brain. 'When they grow and divide, you've got cancer,' he says.

He believes that stem cell research has to some degree diverted funds away from what he thinks is the hard work that needs to be done to find the real causes of the disease and to do something about it.

> *Stem cell therapy is a promise and, like many promises, it hasn't delivered.*
>
> —Professor Garth Nicholson

Professor Malcolm Horne doesn't believe a cure for Parkinson's will rest with stem cells. 'I think they'll be important for symptomatic cures rather than fundamental cures. If we use stem cells to make dopamine then we will only treat the symptoms that come from dopamine loss. We know that Parkinson's disease disturbs many more neurons than the ones that make dopamine. But stem cell research does give us knowledge. They've told us an enormous amount about how neurons are different to other cells in the body.'

Scientist Bryce Vissel says the belief in stem cells as a cure runs the risk of being a rather simplistic idea, because 'the steps between the inception of the idea and its application are going to be fraught with more challenges'. Nonethelesss, he says, 'I think stem cells are a fundamental biological breakthrough. Even if we don't develop therapies, we get to understand more about the development of dopamine cells. All of that is being learnt and that's exciting.' He doesn't believe research in this area is diverting funds away from the field of genetics.

> Stem cells are not going to fix what's happening in the rest of the brain. I believe, for Parkinson's disease, stem cells are never going to be a cure.
>
> —Dr Victor Fung, neurologist

> I don't think the stem cell story is over by any stretch of the imagination. I think there may well be some beneficial results from trials down the track.
>
> —Dr Richard Bittar, neurosurgeon

An Australian–French team of researchers have carried out successful animal experiments using stem cells. They demonstrated that cells found in the roof of the nasal cavity could be used to treat Parkinson's symptoms in rats. The cells produced dopamine when they were transplanted into the brain. None of the transplants led to the formation of tumours, which had happened in another experiment when embryonic stem cells were transplanted into the brains of rats. 'Longer-term studies with a larger number of animals are required to fully assess the risks, but the present result is encouraging, particularly because the rat hosts were immune suppressed' wrote the investigators.

Professor Mackay-Sim told *Australian Doctor* magazine that the nasal cells the team had used normally made new sensory neurons. 'Because they're in the nose, they're accessible. And the other exciting thing is that these cells turn out to be very flexible. They've got a very primitive power to regenerate tissues.'[12]

As research continues to build, experts remain cautious about giving people with Parkinson's disease too much hope. Professor Mackay-Sim says: 'These things are slow. We're right at the beginning.'

> *I think stem cells or cell therapies will happen in the next ten years or so.*
>
> —Dr Meghan Thomas, scientist

In Perth, scientists are trying to turn embryonic brain cells into dopamine-producing neurons in the brain to investigate the interaction between immature cells and the environment in which they mature, to improve the outcomes of this experimental treatment. Dr Meghan Thomas believes cell replacement therapies and strategies to protect dying neurons will help in the future.

> *If we can stop the degenerative process when a person has only lost 51 per cent of their cells that would be a massive improvement. The aim is to prevent the death of remaining cells.*

Stem cell legislation
In Australia, legislation allows stem cell research using excess IVF embryos, but it prohibits reproductive cloning. The re-

search includes somatic cell nuclear transfer (more common-ly known as therapeutic cloning), which was allowed following a review and changes in the law, which came into effect on 12 June 2007.[13]

The states' response to the amended legislation was mixed. Western Australia rejected the move to allow therapeutic clon-ing. Victoria, New South Wales, Queensland, Tasmania, South Australia and the ACT have all passed legislation that mirrors federal laws.

If a researcher wants to use excess human IVF embryos for research, including obtaining new stem cell lines, they must ob-tain a license from the National Health and Medical Research Council. Once created, research using human embryonic stem cells, like adult stem cells, must comply with relevant guide-lines.

The United States is often considered the powerhouse for medical research, largely because of the number of scientists and the amount of money for research provided by government and through philanthropy. The National Institute of Neurologi-cal Disorders and Stroke estimates that $86 million went into Parkinson's disease research in 2008 alone—one of the reasons people have wanted to see researchers allowed to work in stem cell research.

On 9 March 2009, the US president, Barack Obama, signed an executive order ending Bush-era restrictions on using government money for embryonic stem cell research.

Remarks of President Barack Obama

At this moment, the full promise of stem cell research
remains unknown, and it should not be overstated. But
scientists believe these tiny cells may have the potential to
help us understand, and possibly cure, some of our most
devastating diseases and conditions. To regenerate
a severed spinal cord and lift someone from a wheelchair.

To spur insulin production and spare a child from a lifetime of needles. To treat Parkinson's, cancer, heart disease and others that affect millions of Americans and the people who love them.

As a person of faith, I believe we are called to care for each other and work to ease human suffering. I believe we have been given the capacity and will to pursue this research—and the humanity and conscience to do so responsibly.

There is no finish line in the work of science. The race is always with us—the urgent work of giving substance to hope and answering those many bedside prayers, of seeking a day when words like 'terminal' and 'incurable' are finally retired from our vocabulary.

It was an occasion the late Christopher Reeve would have wanted to see, having fought a long campaign to make stem cell research a reality in the United States. It was a fight that actor Michael J. Fox also took on, in the hope that one day it will cure Parkinson's disease.

The dam has broken. Just as I'd hoped.
　　　　—Michael J. Fox, on US stem cell research funding[14]

Gene therapy

Gene therapy is an experimental procedure which involves introducing new genes into the cells of a human body. It's aimed at replacing faulty genes or disarming them, so that diseases can be prevented or treated. New genes can be introduced several ways. They can be inserted into cells that have been removed from the body and then re-introduced. A non-infectious virus can be used to transport the gene to its target or it can be delivered directly into the affected part of the body (for example by infusion or the use of nanoparticles).

Some experts believe gene therapy holds more promise than stem cells.

> *You're implanting a different software program into the*
> *nerve cells. It gets in there by a virus. This is the direction*
> *I think we're going, rather than stem cells.*
> —Professor Robert Iansek, Victorian Comprehensive
> Parkinson's Program

Scientist Dr Meghan Thomas believes strategies to rescue dying brain cells will help patients in the future. One avenue of research involves the use of GDNF (glial cell-derived neurotrophic factor), which is a growth factor or fertiliser for the brain. It is a small protein that promotes the survival of many types of neurons, including those that produce dopamine.[15] Researchers believe GDNF is a good drug candidate for Parkinson's disease after it was shown to increase the survival and growth of brain cells. The challenge has been finding a way of delivering GDNF to a Parkinson's patient to find out how useful it could be. One strategy which has been explored in animals is the use of gene therapy. This involves transferring GDNF using viral vectors: scientists remove the genes in a virus that causes disease and replace them with 'good genes' to invade a human cell.[16] The therapeutic viruses are injected directly into the targeted brain areas, where they release the new genetic material.

Trials in humans have been limited, but experiments on primates show that GDNF stimulates the body to produce GDNF naturally. Experiments to transfer the GDNF gene into monkeys have reduced the rate of death of the cells that produce dopamine.[17]

> *I feel very optimistic about gene therapy. I think it offers*
> *hope in the not too distant future.*
> —Dr Bryce Vissel, scientist

Other proteins also increase the levels of dopamine production, and these could be used as an alternative to drug treatment using levodopa or dopamine agonists. Proteins such as biopterin can also help the process of making dopamine more efficient. Gene therapy would allow the proteins to be delivered inside the appropriate cells to fertilise the brain so more dopamine is produced. Certain proteins or enzymes, including tyrosine hydroxylase and dopa decarboxylase, are produced by the body and play a key role in dopamine production.[18]

Like all treatments, gene therapy carries some risks, including inflammation in the brain. Researchers are investigating those problems and several trials are currently being conducted to test new gene therapies in people who have Parkinson's disease. Much more research needs to be done before this technique is considered an alternative treatment for people with Parkinson's.[19]

Funding research

25 people with Parkinson's are diagnosed every day in Australia. That's expected to treble by 2033 to around 240,000.
—HTA, *Help for Today: Hope for Tomorrow*

In five-year period from 2004 to 2009, the Australian government, through the National Health and Medical Research Council (NHMRC), poured $31 million into research on Parkinson's disease. In 2004, 18 research projects received government funding totalling $1.7 million. By 2009, 31 research projects received grants worth $7.7 million.[20]

Some of the NHMRC-funded projects include:

- a University of Melbourne study into the mechanisms involved in cell death and a possible new therapy to interrupt that process (chief investigator: Dr Robert A. Cherny)

- a University of Queensland study looking at the problems Parkinson's disease patients have in performing more than one task at a time. Researchers will investigate how to best train people who have Parkinson's to dual-task when walking (chief investigator: Dr Sandra G. Brauer)
- a University of Melbourne study looking at home-based rehabilitation to reduce the number of falls and disability among patients who have Parkinson's disease (chief investigator: Professor Meg E. Morris).

A cure for Parkinson's?

Many people with Parkinson's disease remain hopeful that a cure will be found in their lifetime. Some are less optimistic and believe the major breakthroughs won't happen for many decades to come. The question of a cure was raised in interviews with patients, scientists, doctors and allied health professionals. Below is a snapshot of their thoughts and opinions.

The experts' view
Professor Malcolm Horne of the Florey Neuroscience Institutes:

> *When people ask: 'can you tell me what's going to happen in the next five years?' I'm going to say things like: 'at this stage we don't have a treatment that modifies progression. But if you have to have Parkinson's disease, there has never been a better time to have it.' Because when I was a student starting in neurology there were no prospects of a cure. Since 1995, that sentiment has changed. It's not a question as to whether we're able to cure Parkinson's disease any more. It's now just a question of when. That's the optimism I can give people.*

Professor Robert Iansek of the Victorian Comprehensive Parkinson Program:

> *I'm not sure we've got a cure. As time goes by, that concept becomes more complex. I know it lies somewhere in how we prevent the accumulation of proteins in nerve cells, that cause them to die. Where the cure is, I don't know. As far as stem cells are concerned, there is a drive away from that.*

Dr Bryce Vissel of the Garvan Institute:

> *The Parkinson's community, by supporting research, ensure we will bring about new discoveries at the leading edge of a new frontier. We're at a time of great hope. We may be standing at the cusp of a revolution in our understanding of brain repair. This time, right now, provides the chance for a sea change in our approaches to therapeutic development.*

Dr Iracema Leroi, a consultant in old-age psychiatry in the UK:

> *Over the last 20 years researchers have made major advances in Parkinson's research. For the first time, we can say that we are closer to a cure than ever before. However, no two people with Parkinson's will have the same set of symptoms. There is unlikely to be one cure. Instead, there will probably be different cures for different people.*[21]

Dr Meghan Thomas of Edith Cowan University:

> *Understanding the disease pathologies, understanding the different sub-types, is really important because there is not going to be one cure that will help everyone. So if you have different sub-types, you might need a different combination of treatment options.*

Physiotherapist Dr Colleen Canning:

> *I live for the day that there is a cure, and I don't have to*
> *engage in Parkinson's research and look at ways of improving*
> *mobility and quality of life ... then I'll be most happy.*

The patients' and carers' view

Michael J. Fox, the actor and founder of the Michael J Fox Foundation:[22]

> *Christopher Reeve had believed in a formula: optimism +*
> *information = hope*

Paula Argy, young mother diagnosed with Parkinson's in her 20s:

> *I'm really hopeful there's going to be something in my*
> *lifetime, if not my kids'. I'm really hopeful. I'm not bleak and*
> *dim about the future. Even with deep brain stimulation, it's*
> *obviously going to be an option for me and it's only going to*
> *get better. They've refined it. Everything will get better with*
> *science.*

John Silk, diagnosed in his retirement aged 66:

> *I don't think stem cells will help my generation, but the*
> *following one. Everything is heading to a resolution, not*
> *a cure. A resolution in making life easier. To find a cure*
> *you need to make an early diagnosis. There seems to be a*
> *tendency in research that genes have a bigger part to play.*

Pauline England, 73, the wife and carer of Brian, who was diagnosed 20 years ago:

*I always live in hope for a cure. I believed there would be
a cure before Brian got too bad. I've now had to adjust my
thinking and believe the cure will be in the next generation.*

Peter McWilliam, diagnosed with Parkinson's at the age of 50,
and underwent deep brain stimulation:

*I don't think enough is going on. Scientists believe
Parkinson's disease is one of the first ones they'll crack out
of all the chronic illnesses. I'm not sure how close they are.
I still think stem cells are the only hope for us. I'm very
pleased Barack Obama has taken the constraints off public
funding into research. We've been waiting a while and each
year rolls by. The dramatic breakthrough, quite frankly, has
been the deep brain stimulation, but it's not a cure.*

John Ball, author of *Living Well and Running Hard*:

*Maybe there will never be a 'cure' for this disease. My
best guess is that there will never be a single 'cure' for
Parkinson's disease because what we see as Parkinson's
disease may have a variety of causes and therefore need a
variety of cures. Stem cells may be a useful part of a larger
strategy, but I'm not looking to them for 'the cure'. But I
do know that for the first time both the medical/scientific
community and the patient community are working together
to make change. And the biggest change I see is in the
treatment strategy. Rather than treating the deficits in our
motor function, neurologists are treating the whole person
and trying to improve our quality of life. Since my diagnosis
25 years ago, I have seen tremendous changes in both our
understanding and treating of the disease. I can see that our
rate of gaining new knowledge is escalating, and therefore,
I begin to have some confidence that we will find relief from*

Parkinson's disease, if not a true cure. I'd be very happy if that happens in my lifetime, because I don't want my kids to face this, or to face the prospect of caring for me. I believe we are on the right path, but until there is relief we must learn to live better with this challenge.

The journey continues

Paula Argy, diagnosed with Parkinson's in her 20s, now aged 39:

My children are now aged seven and nine, and I have been around to cherish every moment of [their lives]. My priorities are my children and to be well for them. I embrace my life's sole purpose of being their mother. My days now begin much the same way. I am up at the crackers ... the joys of motherhood. I lie in bed waiting for the meds to kick in to bring clarity to the mind and stability to the body. This could take up to an hour, depending on what kind of sleep I have had—insomnia is one of the symptoms of the condition. My two little cherubs greet me with boundless energy. They always have their way of brightening the day. The days are busy with school drop-offs, and pick-ups, ballet lessons, tennis comps, housework, making cupcakes and sewing costumes. I still enjoy organising events but nowadays it's my kids' parties and the various crazy themes they come up with and coordinating the plethora of extra-curricular activities. I am also actively involved in Parkinson's NSW, volunteering at their offices and fundraising.

I have embraced the illness and the lessons it has taught me. I definitely have my moments of weakness when the illness takes control and where things seem so impossible, but I know that this too shall pass. And thus, the good moments are made so much better. On a good day I will be found walking along the ocean. I find the ocean to be extremely grounding and calming even when it's at its fiercest. I have weathered the storm of my illness and survived. The lessons I have learned along the way are ones of appreciation for those who love me unconditionally: my family, friends and my gorgeous girls. There is no judgement in my children's eyes; they love me for being their mummy. When I am struggling through the waves and effects of Parkinson's my mantra has been, 'to just keep swimming' (borrowed from the charming Dory fish in the film Finding Nemo).

FACTS AND FIGURES

Drugs to be used with caution

Parkinson's disease is often associated with co-morbidities. Many medications used for the treatment of other conditions have the potential to alter or interfere with the brain's dopamine system and their detrimental effect on Parkinson's is sometimes overlooked (e.g. increased risk of confusion, hallucinations, postural hypotension and motor disturbances). But the need to effectively treat other medical conditions has to be considered. The following stamp is used to highlight the most commonly encountered medications adversely affecting Parkinson's patients.

NO MAXOLON (METROCLOPRAMIDE) / STEMETL (PROCHLORPERAZINE)
NO HALOPERIDOL / REPERIDONE / PEROICYAZNE

The following charts cover drugs that most commonly cause problems for Parkinson's patients. It is not an exhaustive list: a specialist in Parkinson's disease, or a pharmacist, should be consulted before any medications are taken by Parkinson's patients. Only medications currently available in Australia are included.

The information is from 'Medications to be Given with Caution to People with Parkinson's Disease (For Health Professionals)', 2nd ed., 2007, prepared by Mr Andrew James, consultant pharmacist, in collaboration with Dr B. I. Vieira, consultant physician, and Janet Doherty, Parkinson's nurse specialist. Endorsed by Parkinson's Australia and distributed by Parkinson's Western Australia. Parkinson's WA acknowledges the Rotaract Club of South Perth, WA, for 1st edition.

Levodopa and Dopamine Agonists
Sinemet, Sinemet CR, Madopar, Madopar HBS, Kinson

Medication	Interaction	Action
Baclofen (Lioresal, Clofen)	Increased risk of hallucinations, confusion, headache, nausea and symptoms of PD	Try to avoid combination
Benzodiazepines	Diazepam and nitrazepam may reduce effect of levodopa and increase muscle tone	May be used together but monitor for decline in cognition and symptom control
Anti-emetic drugs (see page 190)	Will oppose effects of levodopa and will make disease worse	Use alternatives such as domperidone (Motillium) or ondansetron (Zofran)
Anti-hypertensive and anti-anginal drugs (see page 190)	May increase hypotensive effect of levodopa	Monitor postural blood pressure
Anti-psychotic drugs (see page 190)	May oppose effect of levodopa and may make disease worse	Avoid the combination or use small doses of Quetiapine or Olanzepine (Seroquel and Zyprexa)
Phenytoin	May reduce effect of levodopa	Monitor closely
Isoniazid	May reduce levodopa concentration in plasma and reduce control of PD	Monitor closely

Bromocriptine (Parlodel, Kripton),
Cabergoline (Cabaser), Pergolide (Permax)

Medication	Interaction	Action
Anti-psychotic drugs (see page 190)	May oppose effects of bromocriptine, cabergoline and pergolide, and may make disease worse	Avoid the combination or use small doses of Quetiapine or Olanzepine (Seroquel and Zyprexa)
Erythromycin	Increases the absorption and decreases the metabolism of bromocriptine	Monitor for signs of dopamine agonist toxicity or choose another antibiotic
Sympathomimetic drugs (cough and cold remedies)	Potential to cause hypertension and seizures	Avoid combination

Amantadine
Symmetrel

Medication	Interaction	Action
Anti-cholinergics	Confusion, hallucinations, nightmares, gastrointestinal disturbances	Avoid combination
Bupropion (Zyban)	As above	Avoid combination

Selegiline
Eldepryl, Selgene

Medication	Interaction	Action
Pethidine	Risk of serotonin syndrome* and other potentially life-threatening reactions	Avoid combination—use morphine

Moclobemide	Increased risk of tyramine-mediated hypertensive episodes	Avoid combination
SSRIs (see opposite)	Risk of serotonin syndrome* and other potentially life-threatening reactions	Avoid combination
Tricyclic anti-depressants	Risk of serotonin syndrome* and other potentially life-threatening reactions	Avoid combination
MAOIs (see opposite)	Hypertensive crisis—potentially life-threatening	Do not give selegiline for two to three weeks after ceasing MAOI
Clozapine	Risk of serotonin syndrome* and other potentially life-threatening reactions	Avoid combination
Dextromethorphan (cough suppressant)	Risk of serotonin syndrome*	Avoid combination

* Serotonin syndrome may exhibit as signs of sweating, high temperature, restlessness, tremor, confusion, myoclonus, ataxia and hyperreflexia.

- Patient's with Parkinson's disease have severe and difficult to treat constipation: caution should be used when prescribing narcotic analgesia, e.g. codeine phosphate, morphine.
- Patient's with Parkinson's disease often have severe and challenging depression: **Tramadol hydrochloride has the potential to interact with SSRIs and lead to increased confusion and delirium.**

Medications associated with drug interactions or worsening of Parkinson's disease symptoms

Antidepressants
Monoamine oxidase inhibitors (MAOIs)

Phenelzine	Nardil		
Moclobemide	Arima, Aurorix, Clobemix Mohexal	Tranylcypromine	Parnate

Tricyclic and Tetracyclin anti-depressants

Amitriptyline	Endep, Tryptanol	Clomipramine	Anafranil, Clopram, Placil
Dothiepin	Dothep, Prothiaden	Doxepin	Deptran, Sinequan
Imipramine	Tofranil, Melipramine	Nortriptyline	Surmontil
Mianserin	Lumin, Tolvon		

Selective Serotonin Re-uptake Inhibitors (SSRIs) and Serotonin-Noradrenaline Re-uptake Inhibitors

Citalopram	Cipramil	Fluvoxamine	Luvox, Faverin
Reboxetine	Edronax	Fluoxetine	Erocap, Lovan, Prozac, Zactin, Auscap

The following drugs from the above group are commonly utilised under specialist supervision

Paroxetine	Aropax, Paxtine	Venlafaxine	Efexor
Mirtazapine	Avanza, Remeron	Sertraline	Zoloft

Antiemetics

Metoclopramide	Maxolon, Pramin	Prochlorperazine	Sternetil, Stemzine

Antipsychotics

Amisulpride	Solian	Chlorpromazine	Largactil
Clozapine	Clopine, Clozanil	Flupenthixol	Fluanxol
Fluphenazine	Anatensol, Modecate	Haloperidol	Serenace
Pericyazine	Neulactil	Pimozide	Orap
Risperidone	Risperdal	Thiothixene	Navane
Thioridazine	Aldazine	Trifluoperazine	Stelazine
Zuclopenthixol	Clopixol		

Antihistamines

Promethazine	Phenergen, Avomine	Methdilazine	Dilosyn
Trimeprazine	Vallergan		

Antihypertensives and Antianginals

Avoid Methyldopa, **Caution** with Calcium Channel antagonists, ACE Inhibitors, Angiotension II Blockers and Imdur.

Others

Bupropion	Zyban	Lithium	Lithicarb, Quilonum SR
Tetrabenzine	Nitoman	Phenytoin	Dilantin

Notes

Chapter 1: Defining Parkinson's Disease

1. Michael J Fox, *Always Looking Up*, Ebury Press, London.
2. Ibid.
3. Parkinson's Disease Society, UK, www.parkinsons.org.uk, accessed 25 October 2009.
4. Centre for Genetic Education, www.genetics.com.au/home.asp, accessed 20 September 2009.
5. *Oxford Medical Dictionary (2003)*, 6th ed., Oxford University Press, Oxford.
6. National Institute of Neurological Disorders & Stroke (NINDS), www.ninds.nih.gov, accessed 2 September 2009.
7. Garvan Institute, www.garvan.org.au, accessed 2 September 2009.
8. Victor Fung, Mariese Hely & John Morris (2003), 'Parkinson's disease and Parkinsonian syndromes', *Australian Doctor*, 14 November 2003.
9. Centre for Genetic Education, www.genetics.com.au/home.asp, accessed 2 September 2009.
10. NINDS, www.ninds.nih.gov, accessed 2 September 2009.
11. Ibid.
12. Centre for Genetic Education, www.genetics.com.au/home.asp, accessed 2 September 2009.
13. DB Hancock et al (2008), 'Pesticide exposure and risk of Parkinson's disease: family-based case-control study', *BioMed Central Neurology*, vol 8, no 6.
14. Department of Environment, Water, Heritage and the Arts, www.environment.gov.au, accessed 20 October 2009.

15. NINDS, www.ninds.nih.gov, accessed 2 September 2009.
16. Parkinson's NSW: Disease Information Sheet 1.7, *PTP and Drug-Induced Parkinson's*, www.parkinsonsnsw.org.au, accessed 25 October 2009.
17. NINDS, www.ninds.nih.gov, accessed 2 September 2009.
18. Ibid.
19. Access Economics (2007), *Living with Parkinson's Disease: Challenges and Positive Steps*, www.accesseconomics.com.au, accessed 18 June 2007.
20. Better Health Victoria, www.betterhealth.vic.gov.au, accessed 20 October 2009.
21. Garvan Institute, www.garvan.org.au, accessed 20 October 2009.
22. Kay Double, Dominic Rowe et al (2003), Identifying the pattern of olfactory deficits in Parkinson disease using the brief smell identification test', *Archives of Neurology*, vol 60, no 4, pp 545–49.
23. Fung, Hely & Morris, 'Parkinson's disease and Parkinsonian syndromes'.
24. NINDS, www.ninds.nih.gov, accessed 2 September 2009.
25. *Oxford Medical Dictionary*.

Chapter 2: Accepting the Diagnosis

1. Fox, *Always Looking Up*.
2. BeyondBlue, www.beyondblue.org.au, accessed 10 October 2009.
3. Pasquale Frisina et al. (2008), 'The effects of antidepressants in Parkinson's disease: a meta-analysis', *International Journal of Neuroscience*, vol 118, issue 5, pp 667–82.
4. *Oxford Medical Dictionary*.
5. BeyondBlue, *A Guide: What Works for Depression*, www.beyondblue.org.au, accessed 28 October 2009.
6. Ibid.
7. G Parker, T Hilton, J Bains & D Hadzi-Pavlovic, *Depression*

Questionnaire, Black Dog Institute, www.blackdoginstitute.org.
au, accessed 15 November 2009.

Chapter 3: Taking Charge of Your Health

1. *Oxford Medical Dictionary*.
2. Parkinson's Australia, www.parkinsons.org.au, accessed 25 November 2009.
3. *Oxford Medical Dictionary*.
4. VSC Fung & JGL Morris (2006), 'Parkinson's disease and other movement disorders', in C Warlow (ed), *The Lancet Handbook of Treatment in Neurology*, Elsevier, London.
5. Ibid.
6. Consumer Medicines Information. National Prescribing Service Ltd, www.nps.org.au, accessed 25 November 2009.
7. Fung & Morris, 'Parkinson's disease and other movement disorders'.
8. Ibid.
9. CW Olanow et al (2009), 'A double-blind, delayed-start trial of rasagiline in Parkinson's disease', *New England Journal of Medicine*, 361, pp 1268–78.
10. NINDS, www.ninds.nih.gov, 20 November 2009.
11. Ibid.
12. Medtronic, www.medtronic.com.au, accessed 1 November 2009.
13. Frances M Weaver et al (2009), 'Bilateral deep brain stimulation vs best medical therapy for patients with advanced Parkinson's disease', *Journal of American Medical Association*, vol 301, no 1, pp 63–73.
14. Medtronic, www.medtronic.com.au, accessed 1 November 2009.
15. Medical Services Advisory Committee (2006), *Deep Brain Stimulation for the Symptoms of Parkinson's Disease*, MSAC Application 1092 Assessment Report, p 10.
16. Rufus Mark, *Gamma Knife Radiosurgery in the Management of*

Parkinson's Disease and Essential Tremor, powerpoint presentation, ww.rufusjmark.com, accessed 17 November 2010.

17. Alan Bensoussan & George Lewith George (2004), 'Complementary medicine research in Australia: a strategy for the future', *Medical Journal of Australia*, vol 181, no 6, pp 331–33.

18. Ibid.

19. John C Coleman (2006), *Stop Parkin' and Start Livin'*, Michelle Anderson Publishing, Melbourne.

20. Parkinson's Victoria, www.parkinsonsvic.org.au, accessed 5 November 2009.

21. European Parkinson's Disease Association, www.epda.eu.com, accessed 5 November 2009.

22. C Stallibrass, P Sissons & C Chalmers (2002), 'Randomised controlled trial of Alexander technique for idiopathic Parkinson's disease', *Clinical Rehabilitation*, vol 16, no 7, pp 695–708.

23. European Parkinson's Disease Association. www.epda.eu.com, accessed 5 November 2009.

24. M Hernandez-Reif, T Field & S Largie (2002), 'Parkinson's symptoms are reduced by massage therapy', *Journal of Bodywork and Movement Therapies*, vol 6, pp 177–82.

25. European Parkinson's Disease Association, www.epda.eu.com, accessed 10 November 2009.

26. Clifford W Shults et al. (2002), 'Effectiveness of coenzyme Q10 in early Parkinson's disease', *Archives of Neurology*, 59, pp 1541–50.

Chapter 4: Stages of Parkinson's

1. Fox, *Always Looking Up*.

2. Abraham Lieberman et al. (1979), 'Dementia in Parkinson's disease', *Annals of Neurology*, vol 16, no 4, pp 355–59.

3. Fung, Hely & Morris, 'Parkinson's disease and Parkinsonian syndromes'.

4. Mariese Hely et al (1999), 'The Sydney Multicentre Study of Parkinson's disease: progression and mortality at 10 years', *Journal*

of *Neurology, Neurosurgery & Psychiatry*, 67, pp 300–307.

5.   NINDS, www.ninds.nih.gov, accessed 10 November 2009.

Chapter 5: Coping with Daily Life

1.   Mark D Latt et al (2009), 'Clinical and physiological assessments for elucidating falls risk in Parkinson's disease', *Movement Disorders*, vol 24, no 9, pp 1280–89.

2.   JA Temlett, PD Thompson (2006), 'Reasons for admission to hospital for Parkinson's disease', *Internal Medicine Journal*, vol 36, no 8, pp 524–26.

3.   Ann Ashburn, Louise Fazakarley et al (2007), 'A randomised controlled trial of a home based exercise programme to reduce the risk of falling among people with Parkinson's disease', *Journal of Neurology, Neurosurgery & Psychiatry*, vol 78, no 7, pp 678–84.

4.   Fung, Hely & Morris, 'Parkinson's disease and Parkinsonian syndromes'.

5.   A Nieuwboer, et al. (2007), 'Cueing training in the home improves gait-related mobility in Parkinson's disease: the RESCUE trial', *Journal of Neurology, Neurosurgery & Psychiatry*, vol 78, no 2, pp 134–40.

6.   ME Hackney & GM Earhart (2008). 'Tai chi improves balance and mobility in people with Parkinson's disease', *Gait & Posture*, vol 28, no 3, pp 456–60.

7.   GM Earhart (2009), 'Dance as therapy for individuals with Parkinson's disease', *European Journal of Physical & Rehabilitation Medicine*, vol 45, no 2, pp 231–38.

8.   Cathy Becker, 'New Parkinson's treatment on two wheels', ABC News America, www.abc.net.go.com, 20 July 2009.

9.   M Morris, R Iansek & B Kirkwood (1995), *Moving Ahead with Parkinson's*, Buscombe Vicprint Ltd, Victoria.

10.   Melanie Tewman, Contact Speech Pathology, interview.

11.   Ibid.

12.   JC Davies, et al. (1994), 'A study of the nutritional status of

elderly patients with Parkinson's disease', *Age & Ageing*, vol 23, no 2, pp 142–45.

13. A Stewart (2001), 'Is weight loss preventable in people with Parkinson's disease?' Poster presentation at the 6th Multi-disciplinary Conference on Parkinson's disease, Melbourne, August 2001.

14. A Stewart, D Long & A Gregoriou (2000), 'Parkinson's disease', A continuing education paper developed on behalf of the Victorian Dietitians in Rehabilitation and Aged Care Special Interest Group, *Australian Journal of Nutrition & Dietetics*, vol 57, no 1 pp 51–53.

15. Parkinson's QLD Inc, www. parkinsons-qld.org.au, accessed 15 November 2009.

16. Ibid.

17. Australian Department of Health & Ageing, www.health.gov.au, accessed 16 November 2009.

18. Department for Families & Communities SA, *Parkinson's Disease: Equipment to Assist with Daily Living*, www.dfc.sa.gov, accessed 10 November 2009.

19. Parkinson's Disease Society, UK, www.parkinsons.org.uk, accessed 10 November 2009.

Chapter 6: Relationships

1. Gila Bronner & Vladimir Royter (2004), 'Sexual dysfunction in Parkinson's disease', *Journal of Sex & Marital Therapy*, vol 30, pp 95–105.

2. Ibid.

3. Ibid.

4. G Bronner (2001), 'Sexual health promotion: an inductive intervention model', *Harefuah*, vol 140, pp 72–76.

5. Lonnie Ali, 'Lonnie Ali's 10 best tips for caregivers', *Readers Digest*, www.readersdigest.com, accessed 15 November 2010.

6. Parkinson's Australia, Fact Sheet 17, *Carers*, www.parkinson. org.au, accessed 5 November 2009.

7. Ibid.

Chapter 7: The Future

1. Solvay Duodopa, www.duodopa.com, accesssed 23 October 2009.
2. Parkinson's Disease Society, UK, 'Four Decades of Discovery'. www.parkinsons.org.uk, accessed 23 October 2009.
3. Health Technology Assessment (HTA) Review, *Help for Today: Hope for Tomorrow*, www.health.gov.au, accessed 21 May 2009.
4. Nikunj K Patel, Puneet Plaha & Steven S Gill (2007), 'Magnetic resonance imaging-directed method for functional neurosurgery using implantable guide tubes', *Neurosurgery*, vol 61, no 5, pp 358–66.
5. NINDS, www.ninds.nih.gov, accessed 23 October 2009.
6. Double, Rowe et al (2003). 'Identifying the pattern of olfactory deficits in Parkinson disease'.
7. Parkinson's Disease Society, UK, 'Four Decades of Discovery'.
8. Karen L Spittler (2009), 'Exploring the causes of Parkinson's disease', *Neurology Reviews*, vol 17, no 7.
9. US Department of Health and Human Services, www.hhs.gov, accessed 16 November 2009.
10. 'Immune cells link to Parkinson's', Parkinson Research Foundation, 27 December 2008, on www.parkinsonresearchfoundation.org, accessed 19 November 2010.
11. Biotechnology Online: Australian Government initiative, www.biotechnologyonline.gov.au, accessed 24 November 2009.
12. Alan Mackay-Sim, 'Promise for Parkinson's', *Australian Doctor*, 12 December 2008.
13. Australian Stem Cell Centre, www.stemcellcentre.edu.au, accessed 23 November 2009.
14. Fox, *Always Looking Up*.
15. John T Slevin, Don M Gash, Charles D. Smith et al (2006), 'Unilateral Intraputaminal Glial Cell Line-Derived Neurotrophic Fac-

tor in Patients with Parkinson Disease: Response to 1 Year Each of Treatment and Withdrawal', *Neurosurgical Focus*, 20 (5).

16. Gene Therapy Net, www.genetherapynet.com, accessed 23 November 2009.

17. DM Gash, Z Zhang, A Ovadia A (1996), 'Functional recovery in parkinsonian monkeys treated with GDNF', *Nature* 380: pp 252–55.

18. Parkinson's Disease Society, UK, www.parkinsons.org.uk, accessed 24 November 2009.

19. Ibid.

20. National Health and Medical Research Council, www.nhmrc.gov.au, accessed 24 November 2009.

21. Parkinson's Disease Society, UK, 'Four Decades of Discovery'.

22. Fox, *Always Looking Up*.

Sources

1. *Oxford Medical Dictionary* (2003), 6th ed., Oxford University Press, Oxford.

2. Parkinson's Disease: Glossary of Terms, www.myDr.com.au.

3. Garvan Institute, www.garvan.org.au.

4. European Parkinson's Disease Association, www.epda.eu.com.

5. National Institute of Neurological Disorders & Stroke (NINDS), www.ninds.nih.gov.

Useful Addresses

Australian Physiotherapy Association
www.physiotherapy.asn.au
(03) 9092 0888

Better Health
www.betterhealth.vic.gov.au

Beyondblue: the national depression initiative
www.beyondblue.org.au
1300 22 4636

Black Dog Institute
www.blackdoginstitute.org.au
(02) 9382 4523

Carers Australia
www.carersaustralia.com.au
1800 242 636

Commonwealth Respite & Carelink Centres
www.commcarelink.health.gov.au
1800 052 222

Dietitians Association of Australia
www.daa.asn.au
1800 812 942

European Parkinson's Disease Association
www.epda.eu.com

Government Assistance enquiries (disability, sickness, carers)
www.centrelink.gov.au
13 27 17

Medicare Australia
www.medicareaustralia.gov.au (information on medical benefits)
13 20 11

Medtronic (deep brain stimulation)
www.medtronic.com.au
1800 668 670

Michael J Fox Foundation
www.michaeljfox.org
1800 708 7644

National Prescribing Service
www.nps.org.au (information on medications)
1300 888 763

Natural Therapy Pages
www.naturaltherapypages.com.au

Nutrition Australia
www.nutritionaustralia.org

Parkinson's Australia
www.parkinsons.org.au
1800 644 189

GLOSSARY OF TERMS

Ablative neurosurgery: Destroys a selected region of the brain.

Acetylcholine: The chemical messenger (neurotransmitter) released by nerve fibres.

Action tremor: A tremor that develops or increases when limbs or body are moving voluntarily.

Activin A: A molecule released from nerve cells.

Acupuncture: A form of traditional Chinese medicine involving the insertion of ultra-fine metal needles into carefully chosen points on the body.

Agonist: A chemical or drug that enhances neurotransmitter activity.

Akinesia: Slowness or absence of muscle movements. A loss of normal muscle response.

Alexander technique: Teaches the best use of the body in daily activities to improve posture and balance.

Alpha-synuclein: A protein prominently expressed in the central nervous system. Clumps can form brain lesions which are hallmarks of some neurodegenerative disease such as Parkinson's. The gene for Alpha-Synuclein is called SNCA.

Amantadine: A drug (e.g. Symmetrel) that causes an increase in dopamine release in the brain. It is also an antiviral drug that prevents the penetration of a virus into a host cell.

Antagonist: A substance that diminishes neurotransmitter activity.

Anticholinergic: A substance that opposes the naturally occurring chemical messenger called acetylcholine.

Antioxidant: An agent that prevents the loss of oxygen in chemical reactions.

Artane: A brand of anticholinergic drug.

Ataxia: Loss of co-ordination in a person's movement, and shaking.

Athetosis: Slow, writhing or twisting, involuntary movements of the arms, head or legs.

Autonomic nervous system: The part of the nervous system that regulates involuntary vital function, including the activity of the cardiac muscle (heart), smooth muscle (e.g. uterus) and glands (e.g. adrenal).

Axon: The long, hair-like extension of a nerve cell that carries a message to another nerve cell.

Basal ganglia: The large grey masses in the base of the brain that are concerned with the regulation of normal movements at a subconscious level.

Blood-brain barrier: The membrane that separates the blood from brain cells. It is also the mechanism that controls the movement of molecules from the blood to cerebrospinal fluid and the tissue surrounding the brain.

Benign essential tremor: A condition characterised by tremor in the hands, head, vocal chords and, at times, other parts of the body—it is sometimes mistaken for Parkinson's disease.

Bilateral: Both sides of the brain (targeted in deep brain stimulation treatment).

Bradykinesia: Slowness in initiating and executing movement and difficulty in performing repetitive movements.

Bromocriptine: A dopamine agonist drug (e.g. Parlodel).

Carbidopa: A drug that prevents the breakdown of levodopa in the body before it reaches the brain. In combination with levodopa it allows more levodopa to reach the brain, where it is converted into dopamine.

Chorea: Abnormal jerky, rapid involuntary movements of the body.

Complementary therapies: Non-conventional health treatments.

COMT inhibitors: Given in combination with levodopa to enhance the delivery levodopa to the brain.

CT scan: Computerised tomography, a form of X-ray.

Decarboxylase inhibitor: A drug that hinders the conversion of dopa to dopamine.

Deep brain stimulation: A reversible operation that uses small electric impulses to block the brain signals that cause tremor.

Dendrite: A thread-like extension of a nerve cell that serves as an antenna to receive messages from the axon of other nerve cells.

DOPA: A short name for dihydroxyphenylalanine, an amino acid that acts as a neurotransmitter, specially associated with dopamine.

Dopa decarboxylase: An enzyme found in nerve tissue and blood, it controls conversion of DOPA to dopamine.

Dopa decarboxylase inhibitors: Drugs (e.g. carbidopa) that block the conversion of levodopa to dopamine outside the brain (so that more DOPA can reach the brain).

Dopamine: A chemical produced by the brain that acts as a messenger transmitting impulses from one nerve cell to the next. It governs actions of movement, balance and walking. It is deficient in Parkinson's patients.

Dopamine agonist: A drug that mimics the effects of dopamine and stimulates the dopamine receptors.

Dysarthria: Difficult, poorly articulated speech, sometimes slurred.

Dyskinesia: An impairment of the ability to execute voluntary movements.

Dysphagia: Difficulty in swallowing.

Dystonia: Slow, twisting or writhing involuntary movements.

Embryonic stem cells: Cells that are capable of producing different cell types required by the developing embryo.

Encephalopathy: Disease of the brain. People who developed encephalopathy during the 1918 Spanish flu epidemic, experienced Parkinson's like symptoms.

Enzyme: A substance that speeds up a chemical reaction.

Extrapyramidal system: The system of nerve cells, nerve tracks and pathways that connects the cerebral cortex, basal ganglia, thalamus, cerebellum, reticular formation and spinal neurones. It is responsible for the regulation of reflex movements such as balance and walking. The extrapyramidal system is damaged in Parkinson's disease.

Free radicals: Molecules that damage membranes, proteins, DNA, and other parts of the cell. This damage is often referred to as oxidative stress.

Freezing: Temporary, involuntary inability to move.

Frontal cortex: Part of the brain where it's thought higher-level thinking and planning takes place.

GDNF: A small protein that promotes the survival of many types of neurons.

Globus pallidus internus (GPi): A structure of the brain that is targeted in deep brain stimulation treatment.

Homeopathy: A gentle holistic therapy to stimulate the body's own healing power.

Idiopathic: A disease of unknown origin or without apparent cause.

Lee Silverman Voice Treatment (LSVT): A technique for improving the voice volume of patients who have Parkinson's disease and other neurological disorders.

Levodopa (L-dopa): A compound that occurs naturally in the body and brain. It is a particularly effective anti-Parkinson's drug that is converted to dopamine in the brain.

Lewy bodies: Abnormal spheres found in nerve cells and considered to be a marker for both Parkinson's disease and dementia. They are found in the nerve cells of the cortex and the basal ganglia in the brain.

Micrographia: Change in handwriting where script becomes small.

Monoamine oxidase inhibitors (MAOI): Drugs that enhance the effect of certain chemical transmitters, such as dopamine, by inhibiting the function of enzymes that break the neurotransmitters down.

MPTP: A toxic chemical produced in making a synthetic narcotic. MPTP destroys the cells of the substantia nigra and produces a condition that leads to Parkinson's like symptoms.

MRI: Magnetic resonance imaging, a diagnostic technique.

Neuron: A nerve cell.

Neurotransmitter: A chemical messenger produced in nerve cells and permitting communication from the brain to other parts of the body.

Norepinephrine: A chemical transmitter involved in governing the involuntary nervous system.

'Off': *See* 'On-off phenomena'.

Olfactory nerve: The special sensory nerve of smell affected in Parkinson's disease.

'On-off' phenomena: A term used to describe abrupt and often unpredictable changes in the clinical state of a patient with Parkinson's disease. It is associated with the effects of the drugs 'wearing off'. A patient might describe themselves as 'on' when the drugs are working, and 'off' when they aren't and symptoms reappear.

Orthostatic hypotension: A rapid decrease in blood pressure caused by standing up. It may cause fainting.

Pallidotomy: A type of ablative surgery of the brain sometimes performed to reduce symptoms of bradykinesia, rigidity and drug-induced side-effects.

Palsy: Paralysis of a muscle or group of muscles.

Parkinsonism: A clinical state characterised by tremor, rigidity, difficulty in initiating movements, stooped posture and shuffling gait.

Parkin gene: Mutations of this gene are the most frequent cause of early onset autosomal recessive parkinsonism.

Parlodel (bromocriptine): A dopamine agonist drug.

Passive movement: Movement not brought about by a patient's own efforts. Passive movements are undertaken by manipulation by a doctor (or physiotherapist) to assist in maintaining muscle function.

PEG: Percutaneous endoscopic gastrostomy. Feeding tube through the stomach. Required when advanced Parkinson's patients become malnourished.

Pergolide: A dopamine agonist drug (e.g. Permax).

Pilates: Low-impact exercise regime that focuses on building strong core muscles.

Postural hypotension: A drop in blood pressure when standing up, causing the person to feel light-headed and dizzy. In severe cases it can cause falls or blackouts.

Reflexology: A therapy that uses pressure on reflex points on the feet or hands to release blockages and to restore free flow of energy.

Resting tremor: Shaking of the limb(s) or body while the body is at rest.

Restless legs syndrome: Restlessness is felt in the calves of the legs when sitting or lying down, especially in bed at night.

Rigidity: Increased resistance to the passive movement of a limb. When the problem is constant it is known as 'lead pipe rigidity'.

Selegiline: A drug that inhibits the enzyme that destroys dopamine (e.g. Eldepryl). It has been used in an effort to smooth the response to levodopa.

Serotonin: A chemical in the brain that acts as a neurotransmitter. The levels of serotonin in the brain are believed to influence mood.

Sinemet: A drug made up of a combination of an inhibitor (carbidopa) with levodopa. The carbidopa blocks the conversion of levodopa to dopamine outside the brain.

Sinemet CR: A slow-release form of Sinemet.

SPECT scan: Single Photon Emission Computed Tomography scan. A type of nuclear imaging test that shows how blood flows to tissues and organs.

Striatum: An area of the brain that controls movement, balance and walking; connects to and receives impulses from the substantia nigra.

Stem cell: Unspecialised cell in the body which can be sourced from early stage embryos, aborted foetuses, blood cells from the umbilical cord and even bone marrow. The cell is able to renew itself and develop into specialised types of cells within the body tissues, such as skin, blood and intestine cells.

Substantia nigra: The area of the brain where cells produce dopamine.

Subthalamic nucleus: A lens-shaped structure in the brain that is stimulated to help treat Parkinson's disease.

Symmetrel (amantadine): A drug that releases dopamine from substantia nigra cells.

Tai chi: An ancient Chinese martial art that combines movement, meditation and breath regulation.

Thalamotomy: A type of ablative surgery of the brain in which a small region of the thalamus (near the centre of the brain) is destroyed.

Thermocoagulation: The use of heat by high frequency electric current. Method used in brain surgery for Parkinson's patients.

Tremor: A rhythmical shaking of a limb, mouth, tongue or other part of the body.

Tricyclic antidepressants: A group of drugs used to treat a variety of symptoms of depression.

'Wearing off' phenomena: Waning of the effect of previously administered levodopa, associated with abrupt changes in a patient's symptoms.

About the Author

Gabriella Rogers (nee Rossitto) has been a journalist for more than 15 years and is the medical reporter for Nine News in Sydney. On the medical round, she has broken numerous stories, including breakthroughs on ovarian tissue transplants, cardiac stem cell therapy, breast cancer screening, and deep brain stimulation for dystonia and Parkinson's patients.

She received recognition from the Public Health Association for her stories on ABC TV in 2000, and in 2009 was highly commended by the country's peak cancer groups in the Luminous Awards for her story on lung cancer.

In 2007, she worked for ABC TV in Sydney where she used freedom of information laws to expose the causes behind the collapse of the Old Pacific Highway on NSW's central coast, that killed a family of five.

Gabriella was born in Perth and in 1992 completed a Bachelor of Arts degree at Curtin University, majoring in journalism and economics. She worked at Ten and News Limited in Sydney in 1992 and returned to Western Australia to become a regional reporter for the Golden West Network, in Bunbury and Kalgoorlie. In 1997, she was recruited by ABC TV in Perth where she developed her passion for health reporting, and several stories earned her recognition from the Public Health Association.

Contributors

This book was compiled with the help of numerous Australian experts who diagnose, treat and care for people with Parkinson's disease. They are listed below. They were all interviewed and gave their own comments with the aim of educating patients, and guiding them in accessing appropriate specialist advice so they rightfully receive the best level of care. Interviews were also carried out with patients and their carers from across Australia.

Special thanks to the following people and their carers for sharing their personal stories: Paula Argy, Pauline England and her husband Brian, Peter McWilliam, Nerissa Mapes, Dan Mongan and his wife Fay, Sue Rance and her husband Phil, Karen Rowland, John Silk and Neil Sligar.

Dr Chris Basten is the principal clinical psychologist at Basten & Associates, in Sydney. He has completed degrees in psychology at the University of New South Wales (Bachelor of Arts) and the University of Sydney (Master of Arts, Master of Psychology, PhD). He is a member of the College of Clinical Psychologists (Australian Psychological Society) and the Australian Association of Cognitive Behaviour Therapy (AACBT). He is a past vice-president of the AACBT. Dr Chris Basten has more than 15 years experience in clinical settings and he is currently a consultant at Westmead Hospital. He lectures postgraduate psychology students and runs training workshops for psychologists on topics such as treating eating disorders and helping people adjust to illness or disability. He has published research articles and presented at conferences.

Anne Beirne is a senior speech pathologist at the Movement Disorders Program at Elsternwick Private Hospital, Victoria.

Associate Professor Richard Bittar is a highly qualified neurosurgeon and researcher. He is a visiting neurosurgeon at Royal Melbourne Hospital, Frankston Hospital (Victoria), St Vincent's Hospital (Sydney) and numerous private hospitals. He is also director of Melbourne's Precision Neurosurgery. His main areas of interest and expertise are surgery for brain tumours, complex spinal surgery and deep brain stimulation. He travelled to Oxford, Britain, to undertake a fellowship in stereotactic and functional neurosurgery, where he worked closely with Professor Tipu Z. Aziz, one of the world's pioneers in this field. Associate Professor Bittar has published more than 40 clinical and scientific papers in peer-reviewed medical journals. He is a member of the Neurosurgical Society of Australasia, the American Society for Stereotactic and Functional Neurosurgery, European Society for Stereotactic and Functional Neurosurgery, and the World Society for Stereotactic and Functional Neurosurgery.

Dr Colleen Canning is a senior lecturer in physiotherapy at the University of Sydney. She is a member of the Movement Disorders Society, Parkinson's NSW, Australian Physiotherapy Association, National Neurology Group of the Australian Physiotherapy Association, the Menzies Memorial Scholars Association and the Stroke Recovery Association.

Deborah England holds a Masters in Analytical Psychology and a graduate diploma in Counselling, as well as a degree in Nursing, and a certificate in Learning and Teaching. She is a Master Practitioner in Neuro Linguistic Programming and is a clinical member of both the Counsellors and Psychotherapists Association (CAPA, NSW) and Psychotherapists and Counsellors Federation of Australia (PACFA). Deborah has worked as a

Specialist Counsellor for Parkinson's NSW for three years.

Dr Victor Fung is a clinical associate professor with the Sydney Medical School, at the University of Sydney, and the director of the Movement Disorders Unit, Department of Neurology, at Westmead Hospital in New South Wales. Dr Fung has a clinical and research interest in Parkinson's disease and movement disorders. He is vice-president of the Movement Disorder Society of Australia and secretary-elect of the Asian & Oceania Section of the International Movement Disorder Society, where he also serves on its Educational Bylaws Committee. He is on the editorial board of the journal *Movement Disorders*. Dr Fung was the founding chairperson of the Movement Disorder Society of Australia Clinical Research and Trials Group from 2001 to 2007 and on the management board of Neuroscience Trials Australia from 2003 to 2007. He is a member of the Parkinson's Australia Scientific Committee and Parkinson's NSW Advisory Board.

Dr Michael Hayes is a staff specialist and consultant neurologist at Concord Hospital, Sydney, New South Wales.

Dr Anne Hillman is an occupational therapist, and lecturer at the University of Sydney. Before joining the university in 1990, Dr Hillman held a number of clinical positions in adult and aged acute care and rehabilitation services. She has published and presented at conferences internationally and nationally, primarily in the area of occupational role performance in later life. Her research interests relate to role, community living and perceived control in the presence of disability. She is a contributor to the ongoing development of the Occupational Performance Model (Australia). Dr Hillman is currently a senior research fellow working on a three-year ARC funded study. Her most recent publication, co-authored with C. Chapparo, is *Living a Meaningful Life with Chronic Illness: A Qualitative Study of Perceived Control and Occupational Role Performance with Couples Living with Parkinson's Disease*, VDM Verlag Dr. Müller, Saarbrücken, 2008.

Professor Malcolm Horne is deputy director of the Florey Neuroscience Institutes in Melbourne, and a consultant neurologist specialising in Parkinson's disease at St Vincent's Hospital, Melbourne. His research interests relate to various facets of Parkinson's disease and related disorders. These include studies into the cause of PD, its genetics, the repair of the brain damaged by PD, and measuring the normal and disordered function of dopamine in the brain. His team of approximately 20 scientists and researchers is mainly funded by the National Health and Medical Research Council (NHMRC).

Professor Robert Iansek is a professor of geriatric neurology at Melbourne's Monash University. He is also director of the Victorian Comprehensive Parkinson Program (VCPP) and director of the Clinical Research Centre for Movement Disorders and Gait at the Kingston Centre in Melbourne. He is the director of the National Parkinson Foundation International Centre of Excellence in Parkinson's Disease in Melbourne, Australia. Professor Iansek is a neurologist by training and has more than 25 years experience in neuro-physiological research, having published over 150 articles, books and videos. He is the recent past-president of the Asian and Oceania section of the Movement Disorders Society.

Margarita Makoutonina is an occupational therapist and a senior clinician in the Victorian Comprehensive Parkinson Program (VCPP). The program is recognised as the National Centre of Excellence in Parkinson's disease. Ms Makoutonina has over 12 years neuro-physiological research experience, having co-authored several published articles. She has lectured at RMIT University and Mayfield Education Institute for nine years. Ms Makoutonina has used her research and lecturing experience to help develop and provide a specific rehabilitation/ multidisciplinary program for people with Parkinson's. She is a member of the Health Professionals Working Group, Movement Disorders Society and has been actively involved in developing their website. Ms Makoutonina has been providing education and training for health professionals, presenting research papers locally, nationally and internationally.

Professor Meg Morris is head of the Melbourne Physiotherapy School at the University of Melbourne. She is a physiotherapist and holds a Bachelor of Applied Science (Physiotherapy) degree from Lincoln Institute and was awarded her Doctorate of Philosophy from La Trobe University in 1996 for a thesis entitled 'The Pathogenesis of Gait Hypokinesia in Parkinson's Disease'. She also holds a Masters of Applied Science (La Trobe University) and Postgraduate Diploma in Gerontology (La Trobe University). She became a fellow of the Australian College of Physiotherapists in 2002. Professor Morris is an internationally renowned expert in physiotherapy, movement rehabilitation and optimising therapy outcomes, particularly relating to patients with musculoskeletal and neurological impairments and disabilities arising from Parkinson's disease, Huntington's disease, stroke, multiple sclerosis, traumatic brain injury and cerebral palsy. She has published more than 150 journal articles, books and other works in the areas of Parkinson's disease, rehabilitation and therapy outcome measures. She is the chief investigator on research projects funded by grants of more than $10 million, including funding from the Michael J. Fox Foundation, the National Health and Medical Research Council and the Victorian Neurotrauma Initiative.

Professor Garth Nicholson is a world leader in neurogenetics, having identified the genes responsible for several neuromuscular disorders. Building on a career of groundbreaking work on the molecular genetics of human hereditary neuropathies, Professor Nicholson's research group has recently discovered new genes and possible new mechanisms in disorders of the spinal cord and peripheral nerves. He has established regional facilities for the investigation, management and research into neurogenetic disorders. These include the Neurogenetics Clinic and the Molecular Medicine diagnostic laboratory, both at Concord Hospital in Sydney, as well as the Northcott Neuroscience Laboratory at Sydney's ANZAC Research Institute. Professor Nicholson's research group, now located in the ANZAC Research Institute, has identified new forms of motor neuropathy and motor neuron disorders.

Deborah Rayfield is a practitioner of Homeopathic Medicine, at the Fountain Centre, Sydney.

Alison Stewart holds a master of science, a graduate diploma in dietetics and is an accredited practising dietitian. She works in the Movement Disorders Clinic in Melbourne and is the manager of Nutrition and Dietetics at Southern Health's Rehabilitation and Aged Care Services (Kingston Centre). This centre is an internationally recognised specialist referral centre for people who have Parkinson's disease. Dietitians at the centre have developed advice for people with Parkinson's disease and their carers. Alison Stewart has published and presented at conferences nationally, primarily in the area of nutrition issues that affect older people and has presented at seminars on the topic of diet and Parkinson's disease to patients, carers, dietetic students and allied health professionals. She is the author of a number of publications including 'The Parkinson's diet', which was published in *Ageing Agenda* magazine in February 2008.

Melanie Tewman is a Perth-based private speech pathologist who treats people with Parkinson's disease. She has previously worked at the Kingston Centre Movement Disorders Clinic in Melbourne.

Dr Meghan Thomas is a postdoctoral research fellow and director of the Parkinson's Centre (ParkC) at Edith Cowan University in Perth. Her research interests lie in neurodegenerative cell replacement therapies, stem cells and neurogenesis.

Dr Bryce Vissel is a senior research fellow and group leader of the Neuroscience Research Program, at Sydney's Garvan Institute of Medical Research. His areas of interest include Parkinson's disease, neurogenesis, dopaminergic neurons, synaptic function, motor neuron disease and Alzheimer's disease.

Dr Scott Whyte is a clinical associate professor with the Newcastle Medical School, at the University of Newcastle Central Coast Campus, and the director of the Movement Disorders Clinic, and Department of Neurology on the Central Coast of New South Wales. He has worked previously with the Victorian Comprehensive Parkinson Program (VCPP) for Movement Disorders and Gait at the Kingston Centre in Melbourne, and the Concord Multidisciplinary Parkinson's disease clinic. On the Central Coast he has helped develop a community-based multidisciplinary Parkinson's disorders assessment and therapy team, and hospital-based movement disorders multidisciplinary clinic. He is a member of the Parkinson's NSW Advisory Board.

INDEX